AF791045

Preparing For Birth: Mothers

Background notes for Pre-natal Classes

Andrea Robertson

ACE Graphics

Contents

How to use this book

This book has been written as a simple, concise guide to pregnancy, birth and the new baby. It has been designed to serve as background notes for the information provided in pre-natal classes and as a reminder for the exercises that your childbirth educator will show you.

A companion volume, Preparing For Birth: Fathers, contains information for your partner. Use the books together as a basis for making this pregnancy and birth uniquely yours.

As you read through the material in this book you will find that it emphasises your involvement in the birth and your active participation in labour. Many women today want to be free to give birth using their own ability and resources rather that just being delivered of a baby.

You are only going to give birth to this baby once, so take your time to enjoy the discoveries of pregnancy and the richness that birth can bring to your life as a woman. Best wishes for a healthy pregnancy, a happy birth experience and a wonderful time with your new baby.

Andrea Robertson

Your pregnancy

Your pregnancy

Eating wisely in pregnancy

Now you are pregnant, you have an increased need for energy to help the baby grow and to fulfil your own needs as your body changes in response to pregnancy. These energy needs increase gradually over the nine months, and during the last six months when the baby is growing more rapidly an additional 700 kilojoules (160 calories) may be needed each day. This represents about a 10% increase from your non-pregnant state. The additional energy, protein, vitamins and minerals required can easily be provided through a healthy diet, and supplements should not be necessary.

Including quality snacks and eating smaller, more frequent meals will help reduce nausea and heartburn and ensure you are getting the extra food you need. Avoid processed and ready–prepared foods which are high in salt, sugar and fats. Try substituting whole foods (cereals, breads, etc) and fresh fruit and vegetables.

In some countries, processed foods such as pate, soft cheeses (Camembert, Brie, blue-vein), raw eggs, raw meat, poultry and ready-cooked meals contain listeria and salmonella bacteria. Either avoid these foods or prepare and cook them thoroughly, as these bacteria can be harmful for your baby.

If you have allergies, take care to avoid any foods that cause problems. You can reduce the chances of your baby developing allergies by planning to breastfeed exclusively for at least the first 6 months.

When you are breastfeeding, you will need to eat extra again, because energy is required to produce milk. You will be making about 600ml of breastmilk each day in the early weeks, increasing to about 1 litre by the time the baby is six months old. The extra energy you will need each day is about 2500–3400 kilojoules (600–800 calories).

PROTEIN

Many women eat enough protein to be adequate without additions, but you should ensure that you have at least 60g of protein if you are small, to about 80g daily if you are tall. If you are not eating meat or dairy products you will need to obtain your protein from a balanced mix of other sources.

The list below gives you some of the sources of protein you could use:

3 pieces of fruit	2–3g	1 bowl porridge	5g
1 potato	2g	2 slices bread	5g
20 peanuts	4g	1/2 cup baked beans	7g
1 egg	6g	1 serving fish	18–28g
30g cheese	8g	1 chicken leg	28g
1 cup milk	8g	1 serving meat	18–33g
1 carton yoghurt	10g		

Vegetable proteins should be mixed with dairy products, for example:

- rice and beans with cheese and milk
- beans and rice, cornmeal, wheat, milk
- wholewheat (bread, noodles) with beans, cheese, milk

CALCIUM

Extra calcium is needed for bone growth and teeth formation of the baby. A total of 1100–1200mg per day of calcium is recommended during pregnancy and breastfeeding, which is about half as much again as is needed by the non-pregnant woman.

Good sources of calcium are:

Dairy products (but not butter), fish (especially with soft edible bones), wholegrain cereals, legumes, beans, eggs, fruit and vegetables.

Three glasses of milk a day will provide 3/4 of your daily calcium needs and nearly half the protein you need. If you are unable to drink milk, or eat milk products, then you should take calcium tablets.

IRON

Pregnant women need extra iron, because extra blood cells are being produced. It is recommended that iron be increased from 12–16mg to 22–36mg daily during the last six months of pregnancy. This extra iron can be obtained from food sources, and may remove the need to take iron tablets, which often cause unwanted side effects, like constipation.

Animal sources provide well absorbed iron:

1 serving of liver (100g)	10mg
1 serving red meat (100g)	4mg
1 serving chicken	2mg
1 serving fish	1–2mg
1 egg	1mg

Plant sources of iron are less well absorbed, but this can be improved by the presence of protein or Vitamin C in the same meal:

1/2 cup baked beans	2mg
6 prunes	2mg
2 slices wholemeal bread	2mg
1/2 cup spinach	2mg

OTHER VITAMINS AND MINERALS

The requirements for most other vitamins and minerals

are increased during pregnancy and, with the generous inclusion of whole grains, fruit and vegetables these additional needs will easily be met.

One exception is folic acid, an essential for blood production. This is found in green leafy vegetables and liver, although it is lost during storage and cooking. Salads are therefore recommended, or lightly cooked broccoli, cauliflower, green beans or brussels sprouts. Alternatively, tablets containing 4mg folic acid can be taken daily instead.

FIBRE

Having extra fibre in your diet will help relieve constipation, which is common in pregnancy. Fibre can be obtained from a wide range of foods, especially wholegrain cereals and bread, legumes and plenty of fresh fruit and vegetables. Bran is a good source of fibre and can be made more palatable by adding it to gravies and casseroles, breakfast cereals and meat loaf or bean dishes.

A SUGGESTED DIET

Breakfast

- wholegrain cereal e.g. muesli, weetbix, wheat germ sprinkled on top and fruit (prunes, apricots) added
- low-fat or whole milk
- wholemeal toast, with a little polyunsaturated margarine
- fresh fruit or unsweetened fruit juice
- 1 egg

Lunch:

- wholemeal roll or sandwich with a filling of salad or fish, cheese, meat or chicken
- fruit
- milk drink or carton of yoghurt

Dinner:

lean meat, fish, chicken or bean dish
salad or cooked vegetables – green and yellow
potato or rice or pasta
fruit – fresh or as part of dessert
milk pudding or low-fat yoghurt
ice-cream sometimes

Snacks:

(morning and afternoon tea, supper)

- wholemeal crackers
- fruit or raw vegetables
- hard cheese
- dried fruit
- nuts
- milk drinks
- yoghurt
- water for thirst

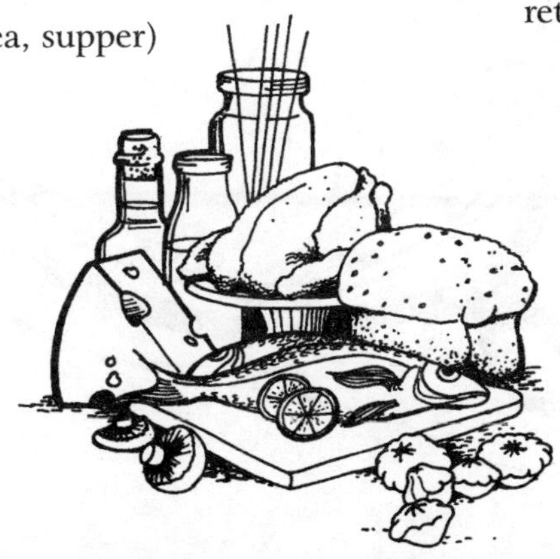

DRUGS

Almost all drugs cross the placenta and many are capable of harming your unborn baby. It is vital that you take no drugs at all during your pregnancy unless they have been specially prescribed for you by a midwife or doctor who knows you are pregnant. Of course, if a particular drug is really necessary for you, then it may be dangerous for your baby if you do not take it as prescribed.

Don't forget that many over-the-counter preparations are drugs which should be avoided unless cleared by your caregiver. Antacids, aspirin, cough mixtures, etc. are some examples. Avoid exposure to chemicals around the house too; insecticides, cleaning agents, garden sprays etc. are all potentially damaging drugs for your unborn baby.

ALCOHOL

For a long time it has been thought that moderate amounts of alcohol would not affect the unborn baby. However, it is now considered that small amounts of alcohol may not be harmful, and those most at risk are babies whose mothers consume alcohol regularly or heavily, on a 'binge'. The only safe stance, therefore, is to avoid alcohol during your pregnancy.

SMOKING

It is well proven that babies of mothers who smoke are at considerable risk of being small-for-dates, born prematurely or stillborn. These babies also have a greater incidence of chest infections and illness in their early years. The more a mother smokes, the greater the risks to her baby. It is now known that side stream smoke from partners or in the work-place has similar effects on the baby, although to a lesser degree than if the mother herself smokes.

MARIJUANA

Research now shows that marijuana may have harmful effects on the unborn baby, and it should be avoided. The problem of passive smoking (being with others who are smoking) is applicable to marijuana as well as cigarettes.

Your baby grows

FIRST TRIMESTER

The first three months of pregnancy are very much a period of adjustment to the idea of having a child, or maybe another child, and also to the physical changes in your body.

Nausea and/or vomiting can be very distressing side-effects of the changing hormone levels and fluctuations in blood-sugar levels. It may help to take tea and sweet biscuits or toast and honey before rising in the morning, and to eat smaller, more frequent meals. Low levels of Vitamin B6 in the system can make this problem worse, and supplements of this vitamin may help. Ginger in any form can sometimes relieve nausea too.

Breast changes. In the early days there can be marked tenderness and tingling of the breasts, with sore nipples and prominent veins as the milk glands develop and the blood supply increases. Nipples also begin to darken. There may be need for a good maternity bra to prevent undue strain on the breast-supporting tissue, and these bras should be fitted by an expert.

Urinary frequency usually ceases to be a problem once the baby has grown up out of the pelvis and the uterus is no longer pressing so directly on the bladder.

Vaginal discharge often increases. If it becomes really excessive, or offensive, it is usually a sign of infection and you should consult your midwife or doctor.

Tiredness and sleepiness are common at this stage, as the body adjusts to all the physical changes involved in the rapid growth of the new body tissues.

By the end of the first three months the uterus begins to rise out of the pelvic cavity and the fundus (top) can be felt about a third of the way between the pubic bone and the navel.

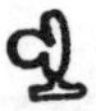

3 weeks

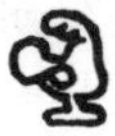

4 weeks

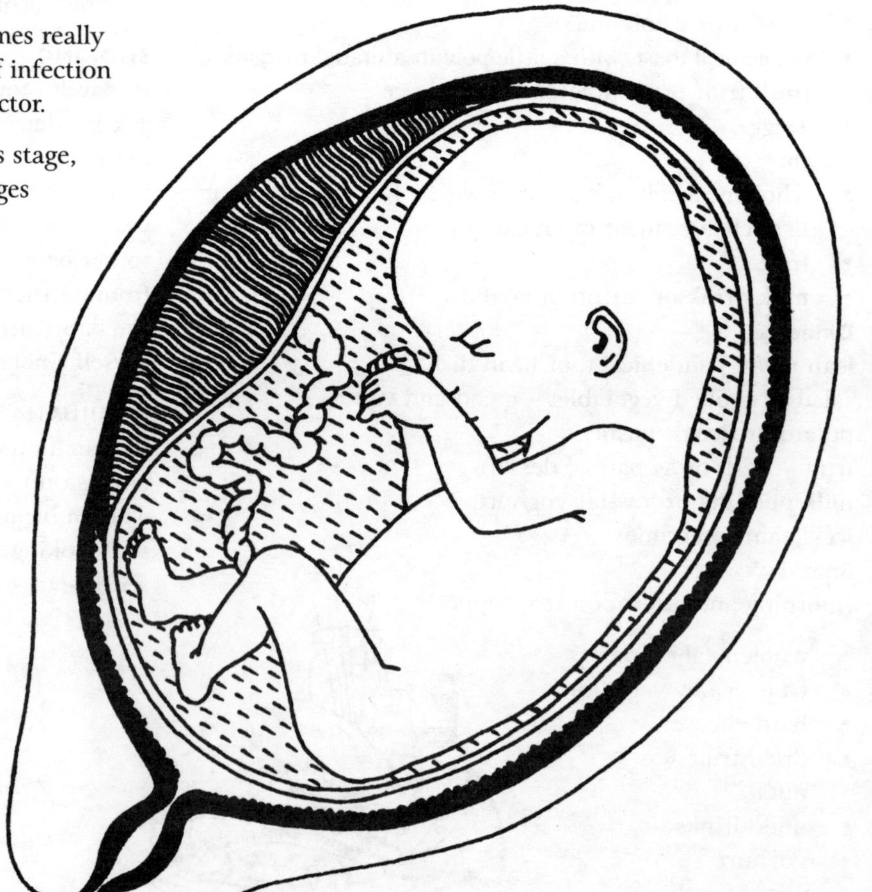

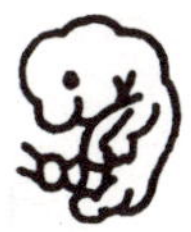

6 weeks

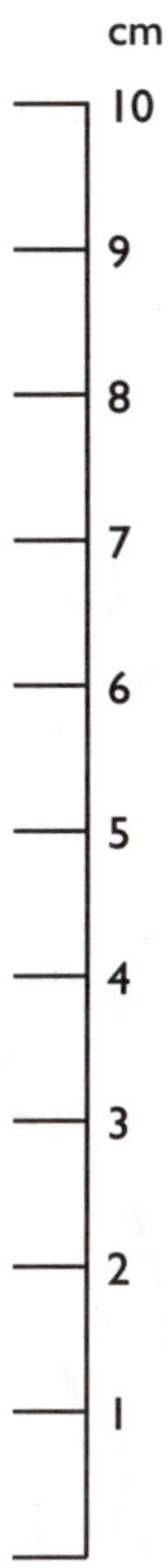

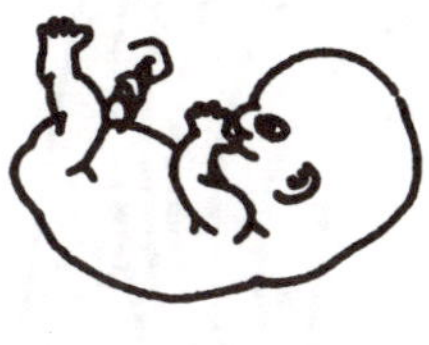

8 weeks

< 12 weeks. The baby lies inside the amniotic sac, floating in the amniotic fluid. The placenta and cord are shown.

SECOND TRIMESTER

The second three months is usually the time of acceptance and planning, and women usually feel wonderful physically, with the whole body working more efficiently. The placenta is now fully formed and operational, taking over the full production of the pregnancy hormones and the uterus and fetus are increasing rapidly in size.

Stretch marks may appear on breasts, thighs and abdomen, especially when there has been very rapid growth, and sometimes the skin feels dry and itchy. This can be helped by rubbing oil (vegetable oil, not mineral oil) into the skin and by not using soap.

Colostrum, the earliest form of breast milk, is secreted from around 16 weeks. It is not necessary to express this, but sometimes it can leak, and if this happens try to keep the nipples clean and dry.

Heartburn, indigestion and constipation are all caused by the increased level of progesterone in the body. This hormone has the effect of slowing down the digestive system, and coupled with increasing pressure from the growing uterus causes these unpleasant side effects. Small frequent meals are easier to deal with and the addition of extra fibre and water to your diet will help constipation.

Urinary infections are common in pregnancy, due again to the action of progesterone on the urinary tract and the resultant incomplete emptying of the bladder. These infections must be treated promptly.

Varicose veins may become noticeable, in the legs, occasionally in the vulva or in the form of haemorrhoids. This is due to the increased laxity of the blood vessel walls (again a side effect of progesterone) and the increasing pressure of the uterus on the veins in the pelvic region. Resting with your legs up may help and support stockings put on first thing in the morning can provide some relief. Vitamin E is thought to be some help, but care must be taken not to exceed the maximum dosage of 60IU/day, as this vitamin is fat soluble and can accumulate in the body.

Backache can be uncomfortable and is caused by the softening of the ligaments in the pelvis and lower back. It is important to try to maintain a good posture with the bottom tucked in and shoulders back. Wearing flat-heeled shoes will help improve posture and avoid excessive pelvic tilting. Rocking the pelvis whilst on hands and knees or resting leaning over a bean bag will ease the ache. See the exercise section for further ideas.

Fetal movements can usually be felt around 18–20 weeks. Sometimes these can be uncomfortable as the baby signals to you from within. Some babies suffer from the hiccups too!

THIRD TRIMESTER

Braxton Hicks contractions usually become more noticeable in the last months of pregnancy. These are usually painless, and come in bouts as the uterus goes through periods of hardening and tightening. These contractions play a role in increasing circulation to the baby, and they are often triggered by activity of some kind by the mother or baby. Towards term they may increase in intensity and frequency and can be mistaken for true labour contractions. A change of activity (for example, lying down if you have been standing or walking) will often cause them to stop and this is one way of distinguishing them from true labour contractions.

Breathlessness and heartburn become more common in the last months as the uterus is at its highest and is pressing right against the diaphragm, ribs and stomach.

'Lightening' usually occurs in the last few weeks of the pregnancy as the pelvic floor muscles relax and the pelvic ligaments soften in response to increased levels of pregnancy hormones. The heartburn and shortness of breath are often relieved as the baby's head descends into the pelvis. Once the head is well down it is said to be 'engaged' and although a common sign that the body is getting ready for birth, some babies don't engage until labour actually begins. This is more often the case with second or subsequent babies.

Urinary frequency is a common symptom of the baby's engaged state, as the baby's head presses firmly on the bladder.

Cramps, muscle and nerve twinges, aching thighs and tired legs are also the result of the increased pressure within the pelvis and direct pressure on the nerves radiating out from the sacral area. Resting with legs elevated may help and swimming is a good exercise at this time.

Emotionally this is a very exciting, uncertain time, as thoughts centre on the coming event. The 'pregnancy amnesia' (caused by increasing levels of endorphin, a natural opiate, in the body) has become part of life and makes it hard to sleep, think straight and concentrate. Emotions are still changeable, with some women finding themselves more withdrawn and introspective and others becoming more irritable.

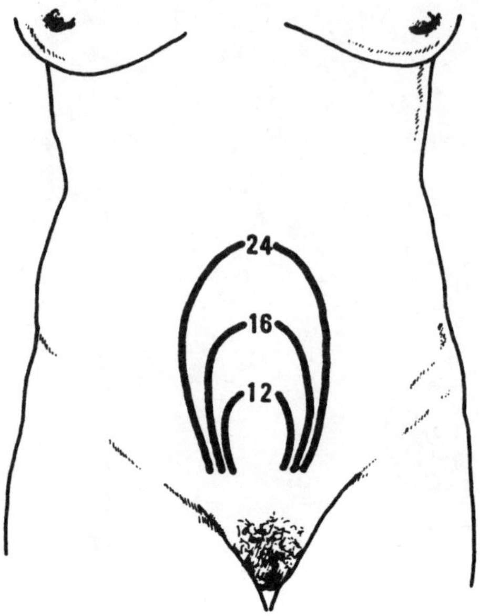

As the baby grows the top of the uterus rises. In the last few weeks, the baby settles into the pelvis (engages) and the top of the uterus lowers slightly.

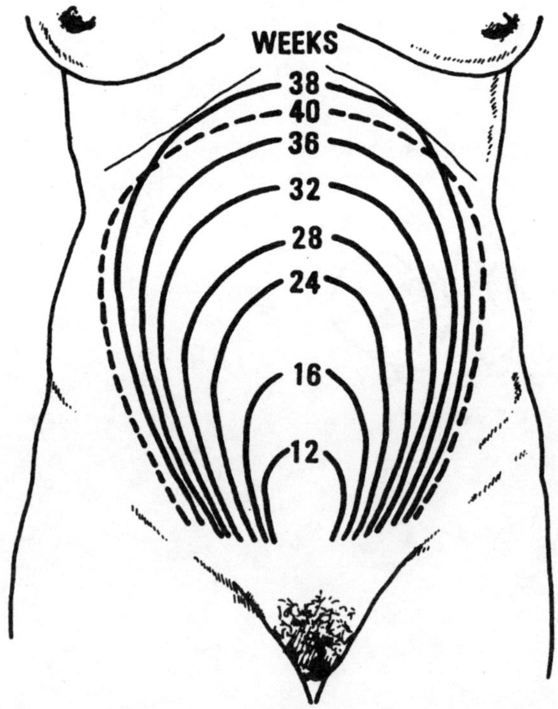

YOUR DUE DATE

It is generally accepted that pregnancy lasts 40 weeks from the time of your last ovulation (approximately 2 weeks after your last period). For many women, however, this is simply not true. Babies who are obviously mature can be born at 38 weeks, and babies showing no signs of post-maturity can be born at 43+ weeks. It is wise to accept that the magic 'estimated date of birth' is at best an approximation; that the baby could arrive sometime before, or sometime after that date. In the great majority of pregnancies, labour will begin when both mother and baby are ready. Ultrasound scans are often used to determine the baby's arrival date and if they are carried out before 20 weeks of pregnancy they are accurate to within a week either side of the estimated date.

If there are any concerns that the baby may be 'overdue', there are a number of specific tests that can be done to determine the health and well-being of the baby. These tests should be done before any attempt is made to induce the birth. Further suggestions about dealing with the problem of 'being overdue' can be found in Preparing For Birth: Fathers.

SLEEP

As the uterus grows larger and the baby becomes more active, it is often increasingly difficult to get sleep. The need to empty the bladder through the night adds to the problem with sleep becoming broken and restless. Towards the end of the pregnancy, the levels of endorphin (the body's natural opiate) rise further and this also makes sleep elusive. Dreams increase in frequency too.

To help you sleep try repositioning your body using extra pillows to take the weight of your legs off the uterus. Lie on your side, as lying on your back will cause a reduced blood supply to the baby and frantic signals from within to try to make you move.

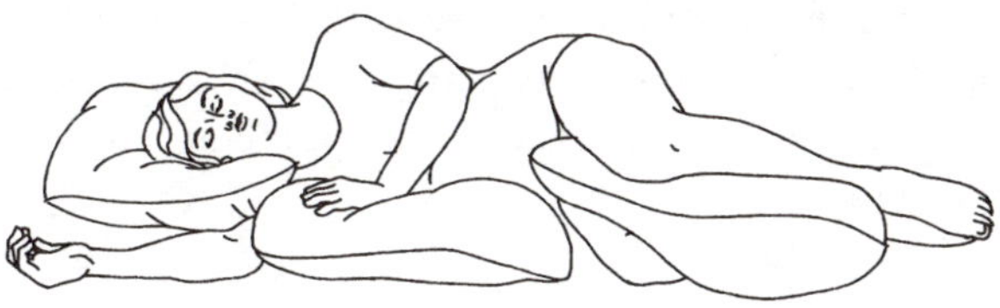

Raising your head and shoulders with extra pillows will help avoid heartburn and indigestion. Chamomile tea before bed may also help. Relaxation exercises, a back rub or stretching before bed may also help relieve tension and make sleep easier.

If you suffer from cramps, try using a pillow at the end of your feet to keep the weight of the bedclothes off your legs. This will help you avoid pointing your toes which frequently triggers severe muscle cramps.

SEXUALITY

There may be completely unexpected changes in sexuality during pregnancy. It is hardly surprising that feelings of nausea and tiredness would reduce the desire for love-making, but apart from this, women do find that their sexual needs change. Some women find that their libido is greatly reduced, whilst others find that this is a time when their desire is more readily aroused because of the increased tissue congestion in the pelvic region. It is important to discuss these feelings with your partner so that changing desires can be accommodated and relationship problems don't arise.

In later pregnancy some experimenting with different positions for sex may be necessary for comfort and this can be a very positive time for sharing the discovery of new and different ways of pleasuring each other.

If there has been a history of miscarriage with a previous pregnancy, you will probably have been warned about avoiding intercourse in the early months at the time when periods would have been due.

It is quite safe to have intercourse right up until the birth provided that it is comfortable and agreeable. Orgasm can cause strong contractions of the pregnant uterus which some women find very uncomfortable, especially towards the end of pregnancy. Having sex will not cause spontaneous labour unless this was about to happen anyway. Some women do use sex to trigger labour if they are overdue and want to avoid an induction.

PREPARING FOR BREASTFEEDING

It is not necessary to strenuously prepare the nipples and breasts for lactation, and no amount of preparation will guarantee that initial tenderness of the nipples will be avoided when you begin to breastfeed. The best way of avoiding problems with breastfeeding is to make sure that the baby is well positioned at the breast and ways of doing this are explained later in the book.

The best preparation for breastfeeding is to allow sun and air on the nipples during pregnancy. Avoid soap when showering as this removes the protective oils secreted by tiny glands in the areola (the dark area) around the nipple. Hand expression of colostrum is not recommended, as it may open the milk ducts to infection. If the breasts leak colostrum, try to keep the nipples dry and avoid protection that traps the moisture next to the skin.

If your nipples are flat or inverted (a very rare condition) the wearing of breast cups inside your bra for some hours each day will help encourage an erect shape. Exercises such as nipple rolling, stretching or pulling have not been shown to have much effect on correcting inverted nipples.

Some women find that as their breasts become heavier, especially towards the end of the pregnancy, a well-fitting nursing bra provides comfort and support. Have these bras fitted by an expert.

Exercise in pregnancy

GENERAL EXERCISE

It is important to continue daily exercise throughout pregnancy. Walking is excellent and should be included in your daily routine. Swimming provides especially good exercise as the body becomes weightless in the water and quite vigorous exercise, using all the main muscle groups, can be done quite easily.

Exercise will help tone up the muscles, increase circulation, and help good posture. It also helps to overcome fatigue and stiffness due to long periods of sitting (a common problem with some work).

Women who have been used to a program of aerobic exercise prior to pregnancy can continue as long as they adjust their exercise program to their capacity and avoid over tiredness or excessive effort. Let your body guide you to a safe level of activity.

Remember to warm up and cool down, and drink extra fluids while you are exercising. Avoid overheating as this can be damaging to the baby.

If you are doing yoga or attending aerobic dancing or exercise classes, be sure to tell your instructor so the exercises can be tailored to your pregnant state.

PRENATAL EXERCISES

Helping your body to become more flexible during pregnancy will make it easier for you to assume whatever positions you find comfortable during labour. You will also become more aware of the way your body works, and find its limitations and capabilities.

These exercises can be started at any time in pregnancy, the earlier the better. Many will help you overcome some of the discomforts of pregnancy, so even if you have only a few weeks before labour you can benefit.

Do the exercises daily. Combine them with some other activity where possible, such as television viewing or reading the newspaper. If you have trouble with backache at work, 10 minutes of stretching exercise during your lunch break may ease your discomfort. Begin by holding each pose for as long as possible (even if only for a few seconds). Gradually increase this time until you can tolerate holding each pose for around 3 minutes.

Finish each exercise session with some pelvic floor exercises, then give yourself a complete rest in a fully supported position as you consciously relax each part of your body. Arise and go refreshed!

PELVIC FLOOR EXERCISES

These exercises are very important for maintaining strong support for all your pelvic organs, especially your uterus and bladder. Learn them now and practise them daily for the rest of your life!

Step 1

Sit forward on your chair and place your feet and knees wide apart. Place your elbows on your knees and lean forward. Your perineal area and vulva should be touching the seat now.

Step 2

Close your eyes, imagine that you want to stop yourself from passing wind or imagine that you have diarrhoea.

Step 3

Now squeeze the muscles tightly around your back and front passages and lift your pelvic floor up and away from the chair.

Step 4

Repeat this squeeze and lift movement with a four second rest in between.

Squeeze and lift several times until you notice the muscles tiring. At first you may only be able to do this exercise 3 or 4 times in succession. With practice, you can aim to improve this number up to 6 or 8 in each set.

Try to do a set of contractions several times each day – perhaps linking them to other activities such as answering the phone, watching television or stopping at red lights while driving.

Exercise in pregnancy - General Stretches

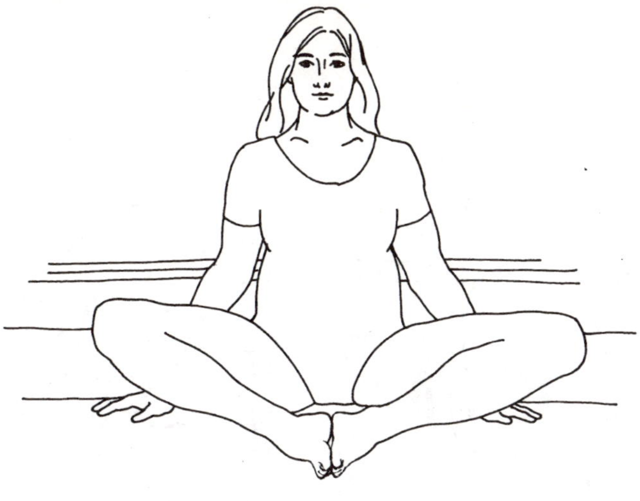

Tailor sitting
Soles of your feet together. Back straight against a wall. Hands either holding feet, or flat on the floor at your sides. Avoid bouncing the knees which can cause injury through overstretching.

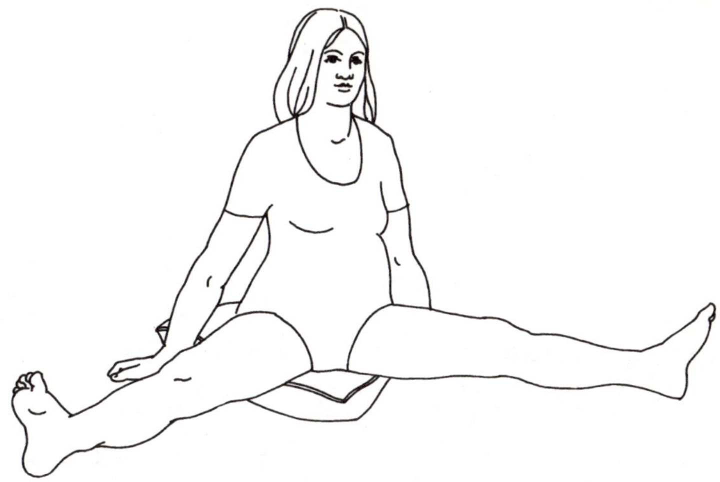

Sitting with legs apart
Sit on the floor with your bottom resting on the corner of a cushion. Spread legs apart with toes upwards. Using your hands at the sides, slide forward off the cushion to give an extra stretch.

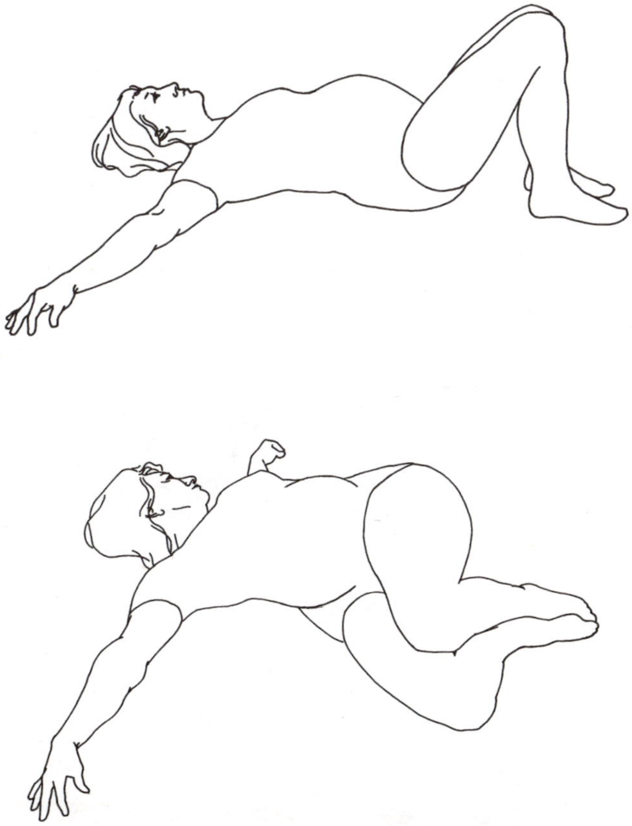

Twisting
Lie on your back, arms outstretched, knees bent. Keeping shoulders flat on the floor, swing knees together to the floor while turning the head in the opposite direction.

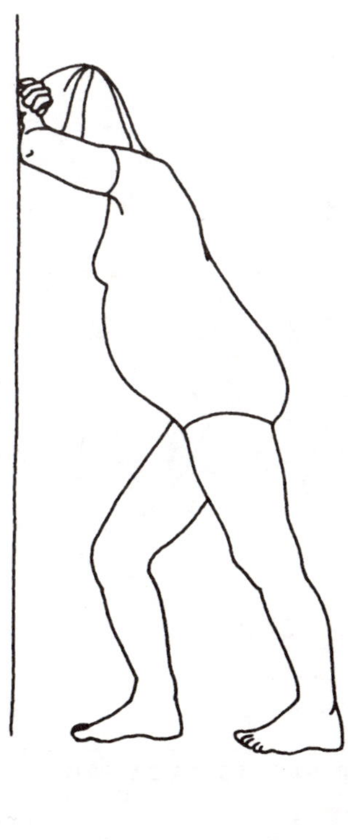

Calf stretches
Lean against the wall, with feet one in front of the other, toes pointing straight ahead. Bend front knee, taking weight on the back leg. Repeat on the other side. A useful exercise if you suffer from cramps in your legs.

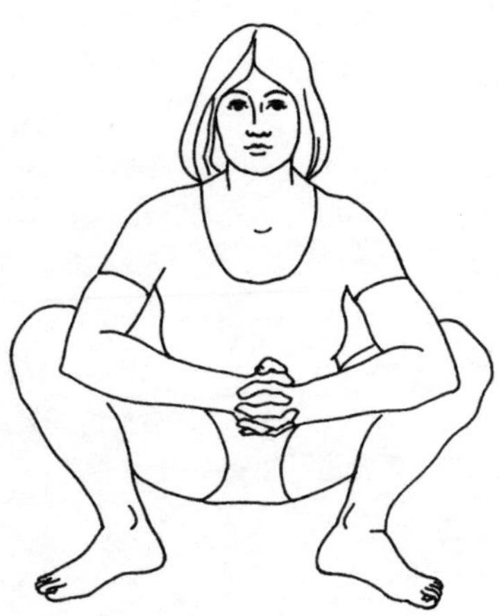

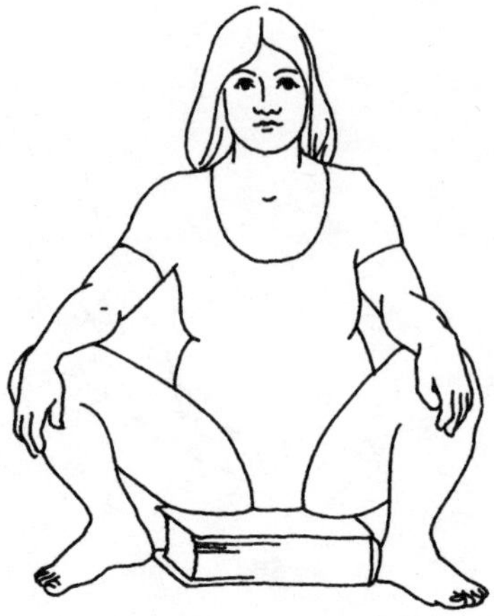

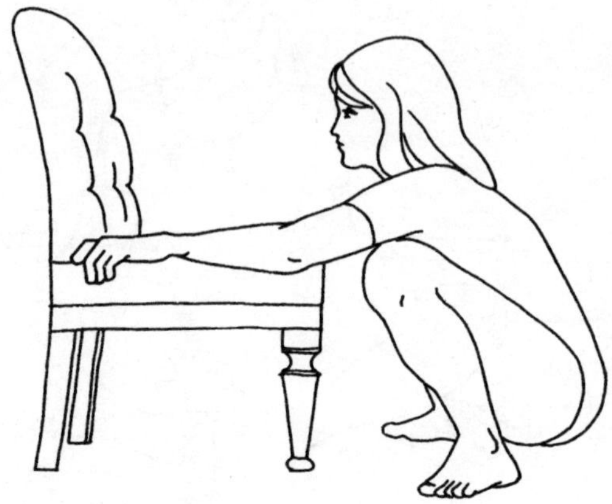

Squatting

Begin by squatting with heels raised and progress to having the feet flat. Pressing knees apart with the elbows will help with maintaining balance.

Try these variations if you find unsupported squatting difficult.

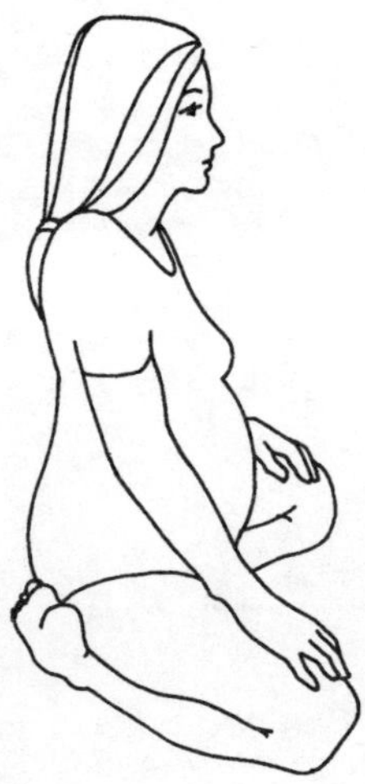

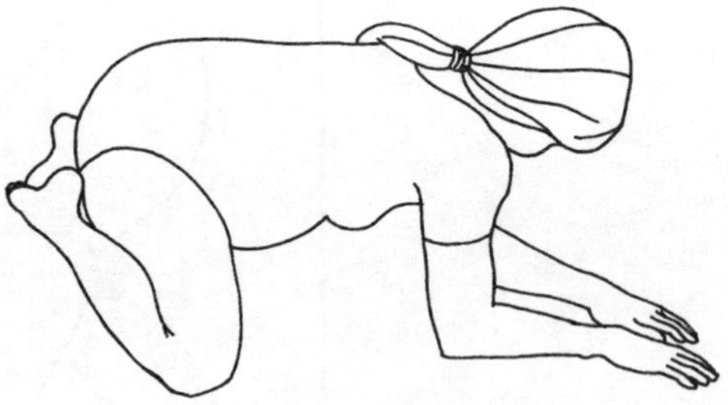

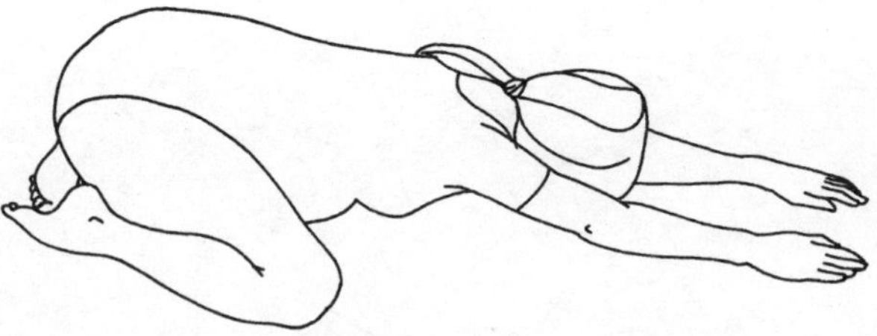

EXERCISES FOR EASING BACK PAIN

Forward stretch

Begin by sitting on your feet, with toes pointed and touching. Bend forward from the hips, stretching arms forward and keeping your back straight. Slide forwards until you can place your elbows on the floor.

Continue to stretch arms forward until your head can rest on the floor, keeping your back straight.

Exercise in pregnancy – General Stretches CONTINUED

Pelvic rocking

This series of exercises is good for easing back ache and for helping the baby into a good position for labour. Begin in a hands and knees position with your knees underneath your hips.

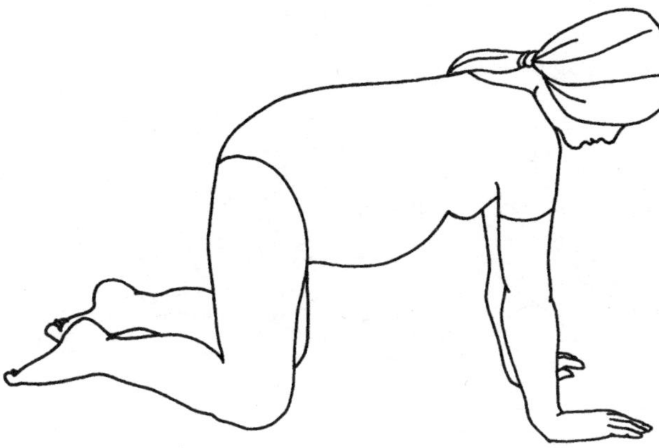

'Cats'

Round your back up then straighten to level. Repeat several times at a moderate pace, to rock your pelvis.

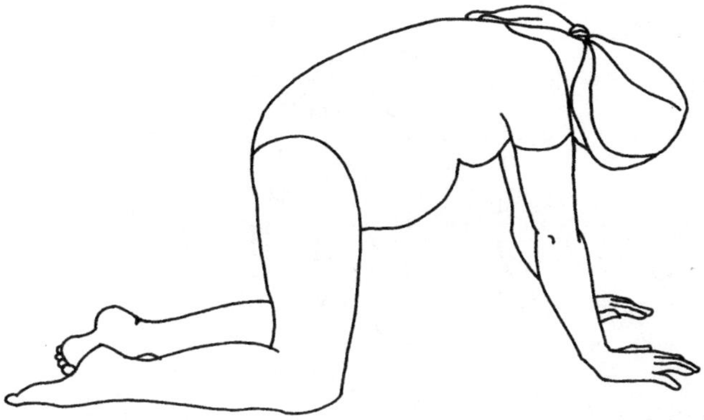

'Cows'

For a sideways stretch, 'wag' your bottom, by turning your head your head towards each hip as you swing it sideways towards your head.

'Belly dancing'

Make circles with your bottom.

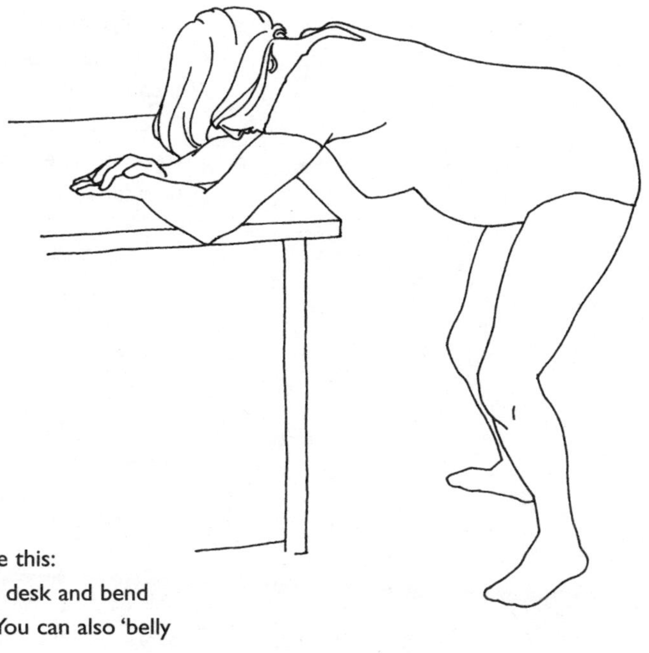

Pelvic rocking while standing

If you have back pain at work, you can ease it like this:
Lean forward with your arms on a table or your desk and bend your knees slightly. Round back, then straighten. You can also 'belly dance' by making circles with your hips.

STRENGTHENING YOUR ABDOMINAL MUSCLES

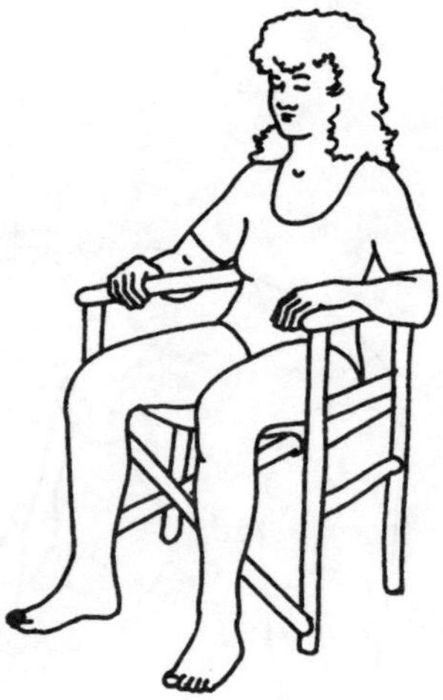

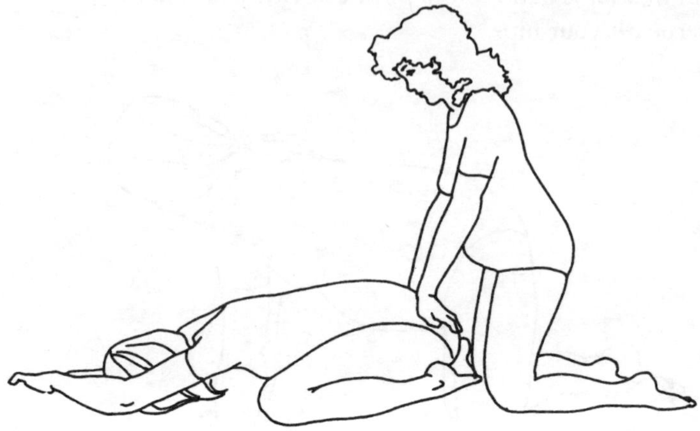

Tummy tucking

Sitting on a chair, pull in your tummy muscles below your belly button, as though you are trying to make them touch your spine. Repeat several times, holding for a few seconds each time. Do this often, and also in preparation for lifting objects or getting up from a chair.

Learning to relax into a stretch

This exercise will help you become familiar with the role relaxation plays in enabling you to cope with the pain of an extended stretch, and simulates the pain felt from the stretching of the cervix during labour.

You will need a partner for this exercise. Avoid jerky movements and excessive strain. Begin by adopting the position shown with your knees wide apart and your partner's hands on your buttocks. As your partner applies gentle pressure, consciously allow your body to 'give in' to the extra stretch, keeping your breathing slow and rhythmical. Imagine your body opening up, and picture the tension easing with each out-breath. Hold for several minutes, and then release.

Practise these extended stretches several times each week towards the end of your pregnancy, and use them as a practice time for labour.

Preparing for labour

PERINEAL MASSAGE

Massaging the perineal area during the last 3–4 weeks of pregnancy will help increase the elasticity of the tissues in this area and accustom you to the stretching sensations of second stage as the baby's head emerges. Perineal massage will not necessarily prevent a tear or the need for episiotomy, but it will help to increase stretchiness and de-sensitise the area to pressure and stretching.

- Begin by lying back and using a mirror to locate the vagina, and the perineum, between the vaginal opening and the anus. Using a natural vegetable oil on your thumbs, insert them 3–4 cms inside the vagina and press the perineum towards the rectum and sides.
- Gently stretch the opening until you feel a slight burning or tingling. Maintain pressure for 2 minutes until the area becomes a little numb. Then slowly massage in the oil, maintaining the stretch and pressure.
- Massage for 3–4 minutes concentrating on any previous episiotomy scars which will be especially inelastic.
- The massage can also be done with a sweeping motion from side to side, with the fingers either moving together in one direction or in opposite directions, according to your preference.

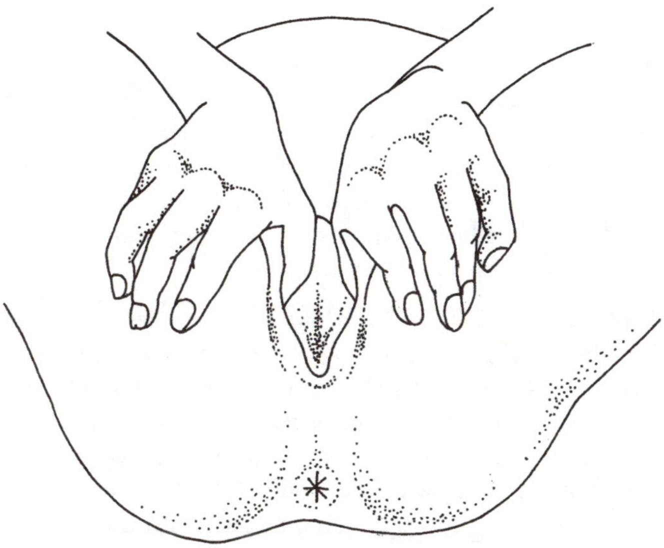

Do this massage once a day during the last 3–4 weeks of your pregnancy.

MAKING THE MOST OF YOUR PELVIS

Your pelvis makes a bony cradle for your baby during the pregnancy. In labour, the baby must move through this bony cradle to be born, and to help make this easy, nature assists in several ways.

The pregnancy hormones help to soften ligaments around joints, making the joints in the pelvis (the pubic joint at the front, and the sacroiliac joints on each side of the spine) more flexible and supple. By assuming an upright posture, leaning forward and taking weight on your open legs, you can increase the internal size of your pelvis by about 28%. This can be helpful in making the birth quicker, easier and less painful.

The bones on the baby's head are designed to over-ride each other slightly as the head is pressed down through the pelvis in labour. This makes the baby's head smaller in diameter, and helps it fit readily through the pelvic bones. The skin on the baby's head will become loose if the head moulds in this way and as it is being born, the scalp may look like a wrinkled walnut! The bones will resume their normal position within a day or two and your baby's head will have the normal rounded shape once more.

Gravity will assist these two processes of moulding and opening of the pelvis. To take full advantage of gravity you need to be in an upright position to make sure the forces are acting in the right direction. Some useful positions are shown in the section on labour.

Using gravity in this way will help you avoid forceps to lift the baby out, and even if you are tired and find pushing hard, gravity, together with your uterine contractions, is often enough to help the baby be born, as long as you are well supported and in a favourable, upright position.

Relaxation

Pregnancy, birth and the early post-partum period can be stressful for new parents. Learning some ways of reducing stress and some specific techniques that can be used to the relieve symptoms is worthwhile. You can practise these techniques with your partner at any time in the pregnancy, and you may also find them helpful after the baby is born.

GENERAL RELAXATION

Find a comfortable position where your body is fully supported, perhaps by sitting and leaning forward over some cushions with your head resting on your folded arms or by being well propped in a comfortable chair with a pillow behind your head. Pay attention to your legs and feet – they should be relaxed and comfortable. Playing some soothing music will help you tune out any nearby distractions.

Take several slow, deep breaths, releasing any tension from your body each time you breathe out. Working from your feet up through your body, imagine each part is getting heavier, looser, sinking into the chair seat or pillows. Continue until you have achieved a state of overall relaxation, allowing yourself time to enjoy the sensation of complete release for several minutes before gradually re-energising through first waggling your feet, then legs and arms.

This general relaxation can be done anywhere provided you can rest your head, and your body is well supported. It can also be useful if you are having trouble falling asleep.

TOUCH RELAXATION

Learn to relax towards your partner's touch. If he sees that you are tense in a particular area, he places his hands warmly and firmly over the part that is tense, then gently strokes from the centre of the body out to the periphery, so that the tension flows out and away. Let yourself go to your partner's touch, so that you are working together as a team. Pay particular attention to areas where tension is commonly felt – the shoulders, back and neck. The face often shows signs of tension during labour, so practise gentle touching on the brow and at the sides of the eyes.

MASSAGE TECHNIQUES FOR LABOUR

There are a number of areas where firm massage can help relieve tension and pain in labour:

Sacral massage: this can be done when you assume various positions.
Thigh massage: for cramps, fatigue or shaking in labour.
Stroking massage: for tense muscles, especially the back.
Effleurage: fingertip massage, good on the abdomen during contractions.

Massage removes toxic by-products of muscle exertions, and eases muscle fatigue. It also reduces muscle tension and can help relieve spontaneous shaking or cramping in labour. Practise massage at least once a week. You may wish to use a vegetable oil to make massaging easier.

Sacral massage is also useful for relieving backache in pregnancy. See Preparing For Birth: Fathers for further ideas on using massage during labour.

USING WATER AND HEAT

A combination of water and heat is very useful for promoting a relaxed state.

In pregnancy, a hot bath or shower will help reduce backache. Local application of heat (flexible hot packs or well-wrung out hot, wet towels) feels good for abdominal aches.

In labour, water and heat combinations (baths, showers or hot, wet towels) are powerful relaxation agents and pain relievers. Check the facilities at your local hospital so you can be prepared. If there is no bathroom available, hot, wet towels are a good substitute and these are also very effective for easing localised pain during labour. Instructions on how to use these effectively are included in Preparing For Birth: Fathers.

BREATHING

Your breath can be used to release tension in labour and help maintain a relaxed state. The rate at which you breathe is an individual one, but try to breathe as slowly as you can at all times. There is no need to learn how to breathe in labour – you already know how to do this and your body will automatically adjust the rate as needed. As the body requires more oxygen and energy, so you will breathe a little faster.

Patterned breathing, or breathing to certain 'levels' within the chest can create a feeling of tension and it is very tiring. This kind of distraction technique often fails to work especially when stronger contractions develop towards the end of first stage. By using a relaxed, deep breathing at your own pace, you will find you can conserve energy and stay calm, in tune with the rhythms of your labouring body.

THE LABOUR ENVIRONMENT

The place you choose for the birth of your baby will have a profound effect on how you feel during labour and how your body reacts. You have an instinctive need for safety and privacy as you give birth, and achieving the best environment is very important for a safe, quick and relatively comfortable labour. Suggestions for setting this up in hospital are included in Preparing For Birth: Fathers.

The people you choose to be with you during labour and birth will also play a significant role is helping you stay calm and unworried. There are a number of decisions you will need to make about where to give birth and which caregiver will best meet your needs. Further information on making these vital decisions can be found in Preparing For Birth: Fathers, as these are issues you will want to work on together.

EXTRA SUPPORT PEOPLE

Research has shown that the continuous presence of a known companion can significantly shorten labour and reduce the need for pain-killing drugs. While many women feel they just want their partner with them during labour, both you and your partner will benefit from an extra pair of hands (or two!) to help provide physical assistance with massage and positional support. Being able to call on an assistant to help with these physical tasks means that the labouring woman can be assured of the comfort she needs at all times.

An extra support person can also provide the labouring woman and her partner with emotional support as well as physical energy. The extra person can take over some of the mundane jobs such as getting drinks and rubbing backs so that the couple can enjoy the emotional experience of giving birth together.

CHOOSING AN EXTRA SUPPORT PERSON

When you are considering whom to invite, choose someone whom you both know well, and in whose presence you feel comfortable. Many labouring women like the emotional support of another woman (especially if she has had a baby herself). Your extra support person could be a relative or friend.

Make sure that this extra person will be available and that their role is clearly defined before labour begins. If you want them to take photos of the birth, make sure they know how to operate the camera. Your extra support person may like to attend your pre-natal classes and see some videos, especially if they have never seen a baby born.

Make sure that you have made all arrangements necessary in advance with your midwife or doctor and the hospital for this extra support person to be present. See page 22 for further ideas.

Medical care in pregnancy

Throughout pregnancy your caregiver will check your health and the growth and development of the baby. A series of visits will be planned according to your needs. Healthy pregnant women need fewer check-ups than those with complications.

ROUTINE TESTS AT EVERY VISIT

Urine specimen – the presence of sugar or protein could indicate a problem.
Blood pressure – the lower (diastolic) reading should not rise more than 20 points above its non-pregnant level.
Abdominal palpation – feeling the baby's position and size.
Baby's heartbeat – after about 16 weeks.
Your weight – although will probably not be weighed, any sudden excessive rise in weight could mean you are retaining fluid.
Swelling beyond the ankles – generalised swelling in the legs, arms or face could indicate fluid retention, a potential problem in late pregnancy.

INTERNAL EXAMINATIONS

A pelvic examination may be done early in the pregnancy to assess its size and the space available for the baby during birth. This examination will only yield approximate measurements, as the pelvic bones can move significantly later in pregnancy due to the influence of the hormones. The only true test of pelvic capacity is to wait and see how the baby moves through during the labour. You can make your pelvis up to 28% larger by assuming a vertical, open position for birth.

A further internal examination may be carried out at the end of the pregnancy to assess the readiness of the cervix for labour, and to determine how far the baby has settled into the pelvis (engaged).

BLOOD TESTS

Your caregiver will arrange for appropriate blood tests, according to your history. Individual midwives and doctors sometimes differ in the number and type of tests they order. Make sure you obtain copies of the results of all tests as this will help you understand what is happening during your pregnancy. Common blood tests in early pregnancy include:

- Blood group and RH factor
- Haemoglobin level
- Rubella antibody level
- Exposure to venereal infection such as syphilis, hepatitis B and possibly AIDS
- Exposure to toxoplasmosis (an infection that can be acquired from contact with cat's faeces).

Medical care in pregnancy CONTINUED

Some of these tests will be repeated towards the end of the pregnancy.

In later pregnancy there are other tests that may be done:

- Triple Test (16–18 weeks) – levels of hormones in the blood are measured to detect developmental abnormalities such as spina bifida and Down's syndrome. Results suggesting these conditions in the baby will be confirmed using either ultrasound or amniocentesis.
- Levels of glucose in the blood (26–28 weeks) – to identify women at greater risk of developing diabetes.
- Continuing levels of haemoglobin (36 weeks) – to check for anaemia.
- Maturation of the baby (36–38 weeks) – levels of oestriol in the blood can be tested over several days to determine if the placenta is functioning well, and if the baby is growing adequately. Useful in detecting small-for-dates babies and to indicate if an induction for being overdue is necessary.

OTHER PREGNANCY TESTS

ULTRASOUND

Ultrasound is commonly used to determine fetal age, and therefore due date. The accuracy of this procedure is increased if the ultrasound is done early in the pregnancy, before 20 weeks, but it still gives only an estimated date.

Ultrasound is also used to confirm a diagnosis of conditions such as twins and an abnormally low-lying placenta. It is also used to confirm the results of blood tests that indicate possible abnormalities, such as Down's syndrome, spina bifida and hydrocephalus. Ultrasound can also be used to measure blood flow to the baby and to determine its sex.

Recent research shows that exposure of babies to repeated ultrasound scans may slow their growth. Until more is known about potential risks of ultrasound, minimal, or no exposure may be wise. Having a scan has not been proven to improve the birth outcome for mother or baby.

The sonic aid or hand held Doppler used to listen to the baby's heart beat uses an ultrasound beam, as does electronic fetal monitoring equipment.

TESTS FOR INFECTION

Vaginal swabs are sometimes carried out to identify potentially harmful bacteria that may infect the baby during birth. If present, treatment with antibiotics during the pregnancy will be recommended.

PELVIMETRY

An ultrasound scan (formerly done with x-rays) is taken to assess the size of the baby and pelvis if disproportion is suspected. The value of this test is questionable, since the picture obtained will provide a series of static measurements and will not show the potential capacity of the pelvis when the woman is upright and using gravity to open her pelvic bones. It is also unable to measure the potential of moulding of the baby's head as it passes through the pelvis.

CARDIOTOCOGRAPH (CTG)

If the woman is overdue or there is concern about the wellbeing of the baby, the baby's responses to uterine contractions can be charted. Using external fetal monitoring equipment in the labour ward, a half-hour tracing is taken, and the movements of the baby in response to contractions (always present, but painless) can be seen. A baby who is at risk will show a slowing of its heart rate every time the uterus contracts, and this may indicate that an induction is necessary.

KICK CHARTS

This is a simple non-invasive test. The mother records the baby's movements during a 12 hour period. She should notice at least 10 kicks in this time. A baby who is at risk will move less often than a healthy baby, with the frequency of movements usually diminishing over a period of a few days.

MORE INVASIVE TESTS

Occasionally, the mother's health or concerns about the baby's well-being may indicate that further specialised tests be carried out.

Having these tests performed is traumatic for many women, who find waiting for the results very emotionally difficult. These tests are not completely reliable, and false positive or negative results can occur.

Before undertaking these tests, seek specialised counselling and consider carefully, in advance, what you will do once the results are known.

Chorionic villus sampling

This is a test for fetal abnormality sometimes offered to women in special risk groups, usually between 9 and 11 weeks of pregnancy. Using ultrasound for guidance, a small sample of tissue at the edge of the placenta (the chorion) is removed and tested to exclude abnormalities in at-risk mothers, such as Downs syndrome, inherited disorders and sex-linked

Medical care in pregnancy
CONTINUED

diseases such as muscular dystrophy and haemophilia.

There is a 1% risk of miscarriage with this procedure, even lower if an experienced practitioner performs the procedure. In about 10% of women , the procedure will be unsuccessful, and will have to be done again.

Results are usually available with 2–3 weeks so an early decision can be made about continuing the pregnancy. Termination, if desired, is easier in the first trimester.

Amniocentesis
In this procedure, the baby and placenta are located using ultrasound, then a long needle is introduced into the amniotic sac and a sample of the fluid is withdrawn.

The test is done at approximately 16 weeks to check for fetal abnormalities, including Down's syndrome and structural problems such as spina bifida. The results take 3–4 weeks to arrive, so if termination is desired it will be late in the pregnancy.

Amniocentesis can also be performed in the last weeks of pregnancy to assess fetal lung maturity and the presence of rhesus antibodies, if the mother is RH-negative.

The risk of miscarriage is about 0.5–1% in the early months, and there is a risk of injury to the baby in the later months, even using ultrasound to monitor the baby's position. The mother may also go into spontaneous labour, or continue to leak amniotic fluid.

Positions of the baby at term

During your pre-natal visits to the midwife or doctor, your tummy will be examined to determine the way the baby is positioned. Ask your caregiver to explain the position of your baby. You may be able to work this out for yourself by judging where you feel the most activity.

The way your baby is lying at the end of your pregnancy will have a major influence on the kind of labour you have and the way the baby is born. When the baby is in an occipito-posterior position, the labour is usually much longer than if the baby is in the occipito-anterior position. Breech babies are sometimes born by Caesarean.

The most common positions for the baby to assume at the end of the pregnancy are:

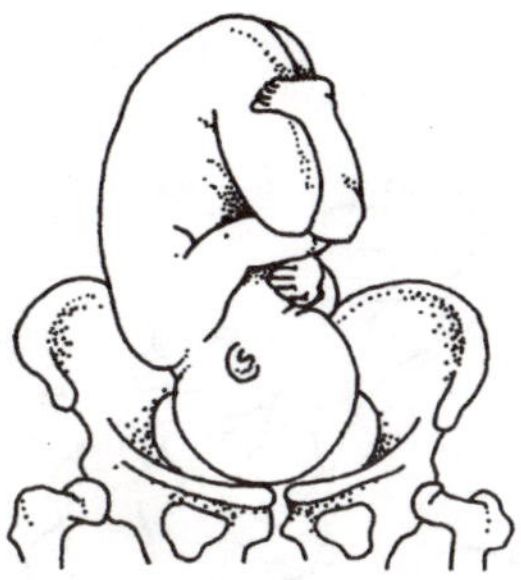

Occipito-transverse
The baby's back is facing towards the mother's side. During labour this baby will usually turn occipito-anterior.

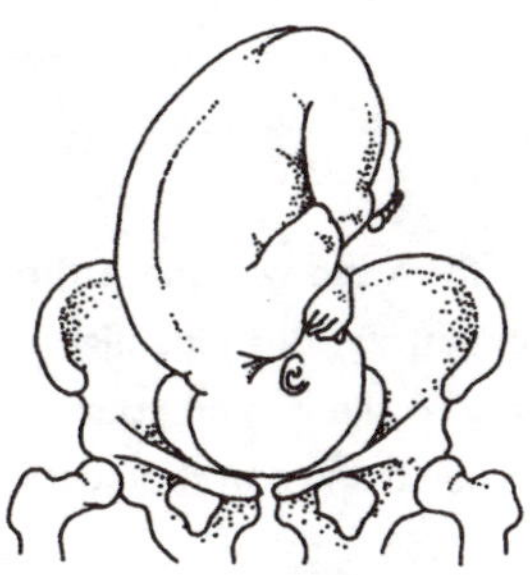

Occipito-anterior
The baby's back is facing towards the mother's front. This is the most favourable position for birth, and the most common.

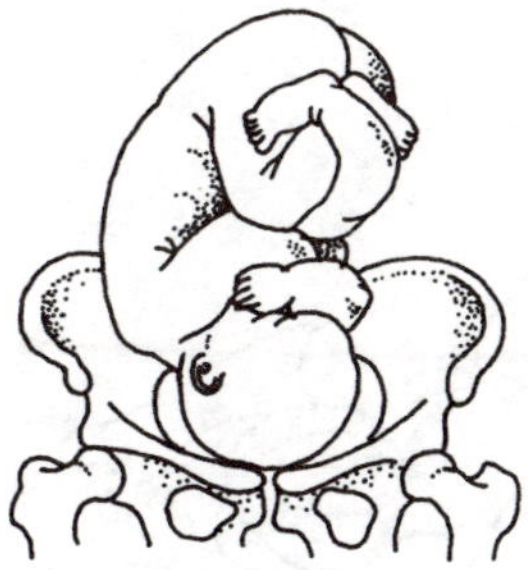

Occipito-posterior
The baby's back is facing towards the mother's spine. This occurs in about 20% of all pregnancies at term. During labour, the baby usually turns to an anterior position to be born. Occasionally (about 2% of all births) the baby does not turn and is born with the face towards the mother's pubic bone.

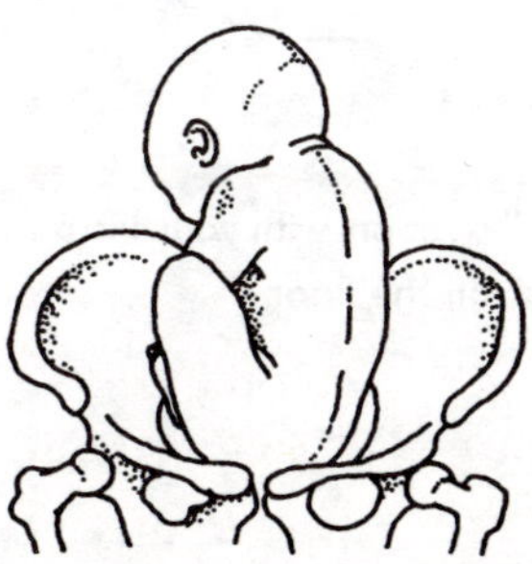

Breech
Only about 2.5% of babies lie in this position.

IF YOUR BABY IS BREECH

Most breech babies will turn naturally before labour. However, to increase the chance of this happening there are several things you can try:

Positioning

If the baby settles (engages) into the pelvis it will be difficult for the baby to turn. This exercise, done 3 times each day for 15 minutes discourages the baby from settling into the pelvis.

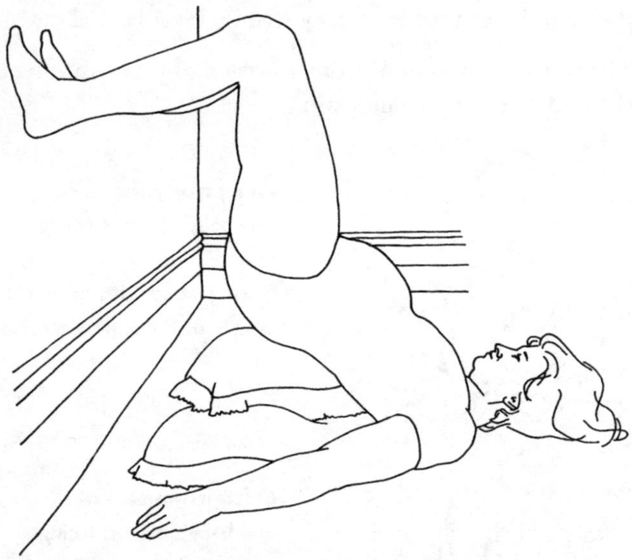

Lie on your back, with your bottom away from the wall. Place the feet high on the wall, and using it for support, lift your hips high. Have pillows or a firmly rolled towel ready to slip behind your back for support. Your hips need to be higher than your shoulders.

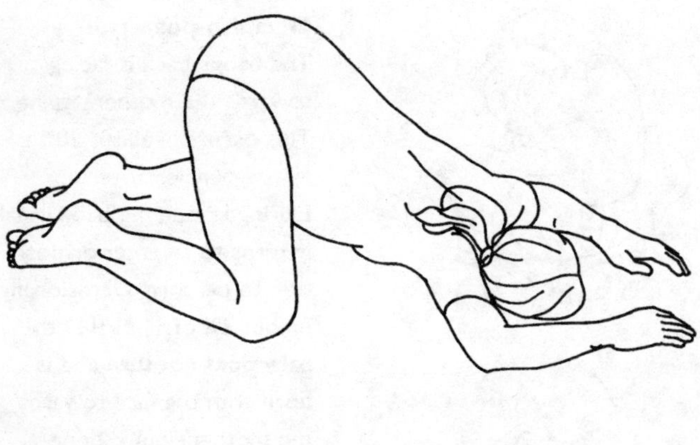

An alternative is to adopt a "knee-chest" position, with your bottom high in the air and your head and chest on the floor.

External cephalic version

Research indicates that manually massaging the baby into a better position is often successful for turning breech babies if done around 39 weeks. You will need to find a caregiver skilled in this procedure, and you may need to take a drug to stop the painless contractions of the uterus while it is being done. As there is always a very slight risk that the cord will be entangled or the placenta starts to separate as the baby is turned, external cephalic version should always be done in a hospital, where a Caesarean section is available in the unlikely event of an emergency.

Complementary therapies

Acupuncture and acupressure can be used to encourage babies to turn from a breech position. You will need to find a skilled practitioner to assist you.

The heat from burning 'moxa' sticks can also be used to stimulate the baby and encourage it to turn. These sticks, shaped like cigars, are available from herbalists. Two sticks will be needed and they can be used several times. Sit on a chair and place each foot on a book with your little toes hanging over the edge. Place each stick on another book with the tip in the gap. Light the sticks (they burn with no flame but an intense heat and pungent smell) and position the hot tip as close as possible to the outside of each little toe, with the heat directed at the point just above the toe nail. Leave in place for 10 minutes.

This is best done just before bed, starting at 34–36 weeks. It takes several hours for the baby to turn, and this will be easier if you are recumbent. Continue over several nights, or until the baby has turned itself.

The research indicates that at approximately 70% of breech babies will turn using this method. If the baby still persists in a breech position, external cephalic version should be attempted just before labour begins.

GIVING BIRTH TO A BREECH BABY

Until recently, Caesarean section was recommended for all breech babies as it was thought this would give better outcomes for the baby. Research now suggests that most breech babies can be born safely vaginally, and that the risk of the Caesarean section to the mother may outweigh any potential risk to the baby from a vaginal birth.

Shop around for a caregiver if your baby is breech. Experience in performing external cephalic version and a willingness to support vaginal birth should be considered.

Deciding on your birth preferences

There are many options and possibilities for labour and birth. By the time you have been through pre-natal classes, read some books, seen some videos and talked to your friends, you will have some idea of the things you would like to have happen during birth and also those things you would like to avoid. Further information can also be found in Preparing For Birth: Fathers.

To help you clarify your ideas, the list below offers a number of possible options. Hospitals vary enormously in the services they offer and the routines they use to manage labour. In many places, you will be encouraged to labour as you wish, and the issues listed below will not arise. However, don't rely on this – it is better to have discussed your ideas in advance than to be disappointed later when your preferences run counter to prevailing hospital routines and protocols.

Assume the pregnancy, labour and birth will be normal, unless there are clear medical indications that a problem has occurred. Go through the list, and note which options you would like (YES) those you don't want (NO) and those options you don't have strong feelings about.

DURING THE PREGNANCY

Choice of caregiver:

______ Independent midwife
______ Hospital based midwife
______ General Practitioner
______ Obstetrician
______ Shared care by midwife and doctor

Place of birth:

______ Home
______ Birth Centre
______ Hospital maternity unit

LABOUR

______ Wearing own clothes
______ Electronic fetal monitoring test trace on admission
______ Consent to be a teaching patient (students and staff present at any time)
______ Returning home if not in established labour
______ Food/fluids on request throughout labour
______ Intravenous drip in labour
______ External fetal monitoring throughout labour
______ Internal fetal monitoring
______ Monitoring fetal heart rate by hand (fetal stethoscope)
______ Freedom to choose positions and activity in labour (walking, sitting, squatting, kneeling, etc.)
______ Vaginal exam for specific medical indication only
______ Full information on risks and benefits of each suggested medical procedure
______ Artificial rupture of the membranes
______ Artificial hormone (oxytocin) to boost contractions or induce labour
______ Access to water pool, shower or bath for pain relief
______ Analgesia or anaesthesia for pain in labour: Kind preferred____________________
______ Partner/chosen person(s) present at all times
______ Siblings present for labour
______ Presence of interpreter

BIRTH

______ Presence of partner/chosen person(s) during actual birth
______ Siblings present for birth
______ Partner/chosen person(s) present for Caesarean birth
______ Birth in same room as labour
______ Position for second stage chosen by mother
______ Pushing begun on mother's urge only
______ No draping of mother with sheets for the birth
______ Anaesthesia for delivery: Kind preferred____________________
______ No specific time limit on second stage if progress is being made
______ Episiotomy
______ Freedom to touch baby during birth
______ Father/mother assisting with actual birth by hand
______ Midwife to assist baby's birth
______ Female rather than male doctor
______ Baby allowed to take first breaths unassisted (no immediate suctioning, etc.)
______ Late cord clamping (after pulsating stops)
______ Skin-to-skin contact for mother and father with baby immediately after birth
______ Artificial hormone injection (oxytocin) after the birth to expel the placenta
______ Baby on breast to stimulate expulsion of placenta
______ Vernix left on
______ Baby weighed, measured in parents' presence after initial bonding period

POST NATAL

______ Baby remains with mother at all times (nights included)
______ Person of choice in mother's room at any time of day
______ Breastfeeding on demand from birth
______ Help with breastfeeding on request
______ Formula feeding
______ Vitamin K for baby: oral / injection/with held unless requested by parents
______ Circumcision
______ Early discharge from hospital as soon as mother wishes

Implementing your birth preferences

It may not be easy to have the birth experience you have planned. Caregivers and hospitals vary in their views and practices, and it is wise to work out your particular requirements early in the pregnancy so you can take steps to find the services you will need in plenty of time for the birth. Details of the options in caregivers and birth place are described in Preparing For Birth: Fathers. You will want to discuss these ideas in detail with your partner and enlist his help in negotiating with hospital staff and caregivers.

Here are some ideas on how you can both go about achieving your goals:

- Find out as much as you can about birth: the process, current practices in hospitals, professional views, etc. Don't just rely on what your friends experienced; ask around widely. Your class teacher will have plenty of information too.
- When you feel ready to make decisions, use this plan to work out what is important to you. There may be some aspects that you will definitely want, or not want, and some areas in which you have no particular strong feelings.
- Discuss your needs with the midwife or doctor as soon as possible. Determine which areas may need further discussion and/or compromise, and those areas in which you agree.
- Visit the hospital and find out their procedures, and how they can meet your needs. Decide if there are areas where compromise will be needed.
- Think about these areas needing compromise. How important are these issues to you? Can you think of any solutions that may be acceptable to all parties?
- Discuss your ideas further with the midwife or doctor and hospital staff. Try to work out mutually acceptable compromises in the areas in which you feel this is needed.
- Look again at your chosen caregiver and birthplace: are there any others who might be willing to accommodate your needs and where compromise will not be needed?
- If you feel you can achieve a happier result with another caregiver or hospital, then consider changing. You can do this even late in pregnancy if you want, and your new caregiver will request your medical notes from your previous one (you could also request these notes yourself).
- If you don't want to change caregivers then you may have to be prepared to accommodate their wishes in certain areas. By deciding early in pregnancy, there will be more time for you to adjust to this, and to explore other ways of redeeming the situation.
- Make sure that both the midwife or doctor and the hospital staff know, well in advance of your labour, what you would like. Visit the hospital again if necessary, to finalise arrangements with the labour ward staff or the post-natal staff. You could also ask your caregiver for a letter outlining the care you want, for you to take with you to the hospital. This way, even if s(he) doesn't make it, or arrives late in labour, you have a chance of getting the experience you have planned. Make sure that this letter from the doctor is attached to your medical notes.
- Check your hospital's consent form: does it allow for informed consent, after consultation, for all procedures or treatments you will be offered?

It is important to remember when going through these steps:

- It may be unreasonable to expect your caregiver to radically change their method of managing births just for you. You might be better off seeking a more sympathetic person.
- It is unreasonable to expect the hospital staff to accede to your wishes if you haven't spoken to them during pregnancy. They may be unable to provide special care if not warned beforehand that you will want it, and they will be understandably hostile if you come to their ward full of demands.
- The most important point of all: caregivers cannot read your mind. Don't be afraid to talk about anything that is bothering you with those who will be caring for you. Don't assume that 'all will be well'; ask and make sure. Then everyone knows where they stand.

After it is all over it is nice to:

- Write to the hospital and doctor and thank them for their care, especially any 'extras' they have provided. It not only lets them know that you were happy with their efforts and thus encourages them, but it helps to set a precedent for others who will follow you.
- If you are unhappy about some aspect of your care, tell the appropriate people that too. They need to know how you felt about their assistance.
- Attend your class reunion to let your classmates know how you went and to give your teacher some feedback.
- Fill in your labour questionnaire and return it.

The birth of your baby

The birth of your baby

Labour begins

SIGNS OF IMPENDING LABOUR

In the last weeks of pregnancy, you may notice some of the following signs that your body and the baby are getting ready for labour:

- The baby's head engages into the pelvis. This happens 2–6 weeks before labour begins, but may not happen until labour starts (especially if this is not your first baby).
- Braxton-Hicks contractions: usually painless tightenings of the uterus, but occurring more often than in the earlier months of pregnancy, perhaps as 'sets' of contractions.
- Increased mucous discharge from the vagina.
- Weight loss of around 500g–1kg in the week before labour begins, due to a reduction of amniotic fluid around the baby.
- Baby may be less active, as it runs out of space and also prepares for the labour to come.
- Spurt of energy in the mother: nesting behaviour.
- Slight diarrhoea.
- Pelvic pressure due to the baby's position low in the pelvis.
- A 'show' of pinky mucous discharge from the vagina, perhaps streaked with blood.
- Waters breaking with no subsequent labour contractions.

HOW WILL YOU KNOW YOU ARE IN LABOUR?

Following some of the signs listed above, contractions will develop. These feel different from the Braxton-Hicks contractions of pregnancy. Labour contractions:

- Have a rhythmic quality, with each one gradually building to a peak and then fading.
- Develop into a pattern of increasing intensity over time. The length of time between each one is less important than the length and strength of the contraction itself.
- Require concentration. You will not want to talk or continue with daily activities.
- Will encourage you to find a comfortable position to ease the pain.
- Are strong enough that you will want to rest in between.
- Sometimes are felt as a constant minor backache, with regular bouts of stronger back pain.

Until the contractions are feeling like this, you are probably not in labour.

Occasionally, the membranes leak or break (about 10–15% of labours). Contractions may start immediately, but often they take hours or even days to become established. Once the symptoms described above are present, you will know that labour truly has begun, and until then you should carry on as usual with your daily life. For further ideas, see Preparing For Birth: Fathers.

WHEN TO GO TO HOSPITAL

During the first part of labour you will be most comfortable at home, in a familiar environment where you can make yourself comfortable. As the contractions become more productive they will begin to settle into a pattern. The best guide to the intensity and strength of contractions is their length, and once they are lasting 60 seconds or more, dilatation will be occurring.

You will know when you feel you need to go to hospital and as soon as you no longer feel comfortable in your own home, then you should ask your partner to take you. It is wise to stay at home as long as possible to avoid many unnecessary hours in the hospital, especially if this is your first baby.

You may be more comfortable travelling on hands and knees on the back seat or sitting on the back seat leaning forward onto the back of the passenger seat, if this can be pushed right forward. See Preparing For Birth: Fathers for more suggestions.

When you get to the hospital, go to the admission desk and complete the formalities. You will be shown to the labour ward by a staff member.

If you are having a home birth you will naturally stay at home and call the midwife when you want her to be with you. In the very unlikely event of a complication, your midwife will indicate when it is appropriate or necessary to go to the hospital.

ADMISSION INTO HOSPITAL

When you arrive in the labour ward, basic observations will be taken: blood pressure, urine check, temperature, obstetric history, pregnancy history. The midwife will listen to the baby's heartbeat and feel its position in the abdomen. An internal examination will be made to assess progress. You can sit on a chair for these examinations, and your partner will be able to stay with you while they are done.

Some hospitals have a policy of recording a 20–30 minute trace on the electronic fetal monitor as part of their admission procedure. There is no need to lie down for this – sitting or standing is healthier for the baby as it reduces the risk of jeopardising the baby's blood supply from lying on your back. There is no research to prove that a benefit in birth outcome results from using routine electronic monitoring in labour.

Labour begins CONTINUED

When these admission procedures are completed you will be shown to your labour room or to the first stage area where you can make yourself comfortable.

Sometimes, labour can slow down when you get to the hospital, and can even stop altogether. If this happens, it is your body's natural reaction to the change of environment. Give yourself time to adjust to the surroundings and the staff. Labour will re-establish when you are feeling comfortable. Alternatively, you might want to go home again, especially if you are in very early labour. The midwife will be able to tell you how dilated you are after she examines you. There is no need to speed up labour that has slowed in this way unless the baby shows clear signs of being distressed, which is rare.

HOW LONG IS LABOUR?

Every mother would like to know how long her labour will be, before she begins. Unfortunately, it is impossible to anticipate how long labour will take, because each woman has her own individual way of giving birth. In general, giving birth to your first baby takes longer than giving birth to subsequent children, but each labour will still vary, and keeping an open mind will help you prepare for all eventualities.

The average length of the first stage of labour with your first baby is from 12–14 hours, and for second stage, from 1–2 hours. Labour and birth can take much longer than this and still be normal and as long as mother and baby are in good health, the length of labour itself need be no cause for concern.

With subsequent births, the average length of first stage is 6–8 hours with second stage taking from 5 minutes to 1 hour to complete.

Remember that your body knows how to give birth, just as your body knows how to grow the baby in the first place. Trust in your instincts and allow yourself time to explore the sensations you will feel. How long it will take depends on many factors, such as your comfort, emotional support, the position of the baby, the position you assume and how you feel about becoming a mother. Having a baby is an adventure into the unknown, but one that is enormously rewarding.

The diagram illustrates the general pattern of labour. It is often difficult to pinpoint when labour has actually begun as there can be quite a long period in which some early warning signs are present, but little other action. This is an outline of an average first labour. There are many variations on this theme, and you will have to wait until the contractions start to discover how your body will undertake the task of giving birth. Be prepared to accept whatever your particular labour brings and allow yourself time to adjust and to appreciate the powerful energy that is yours as you give birth.

MAKING LABOUR EASIER

In general, your body will work best if you feel safe and secure as you labour. This can be achieved through:

- Having the close, continuous support from your partner or close friends or relatives during labour. Having suitable support has been shown to shorten labours and reduce the need for pain killing drugs.
- Finding a place to labour that is dark, quiet and cosy. The labour ward can be altered to provide these conditions: dim the lights, keep the door closed and move the bed to give yourself more floor space for mats, bean bags, chairs etc.
- Stay as vertical as you can to stimulate the labour and make the contractions more comfortable. The positions on the following pages show how this can be done.
- Have regular drinks during labour and eat light snacks in the early stages.
- Stay focused on what you are doing and respond to our instinctive urges as necessary. This is the one time when you can be the complete centre of attention, and your every wish will be readily fulfilled!

Further information on setting up an appropriate labouring environment in the hospital is included in Preparing For Birth: Fathers.

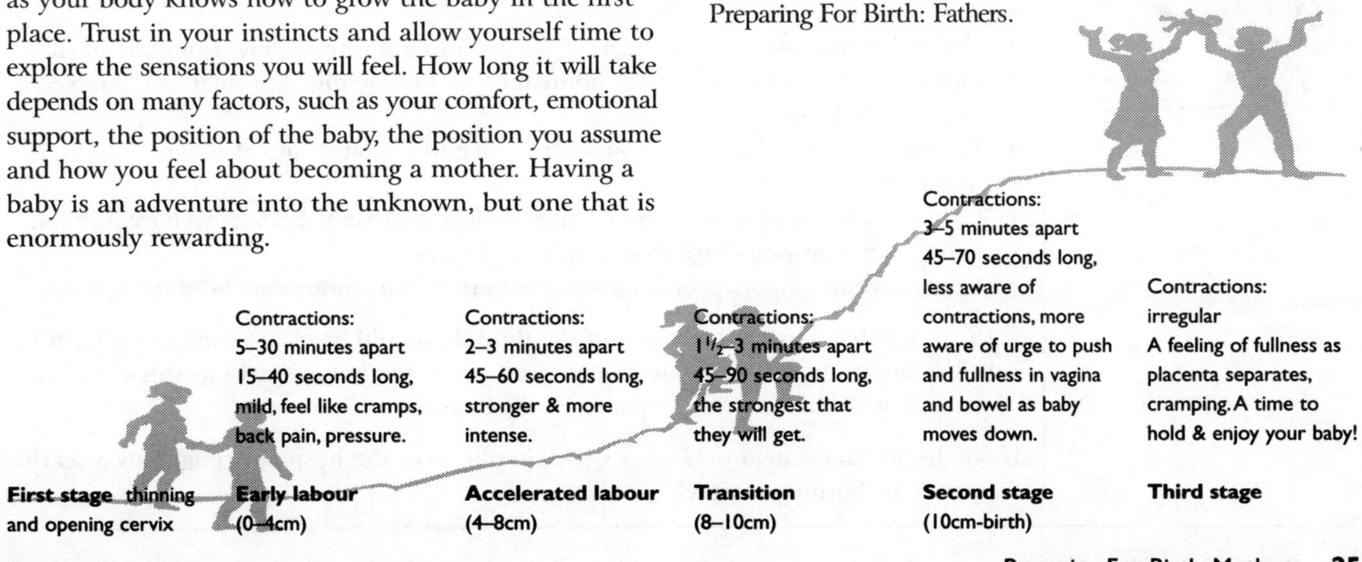

Your labour and birth

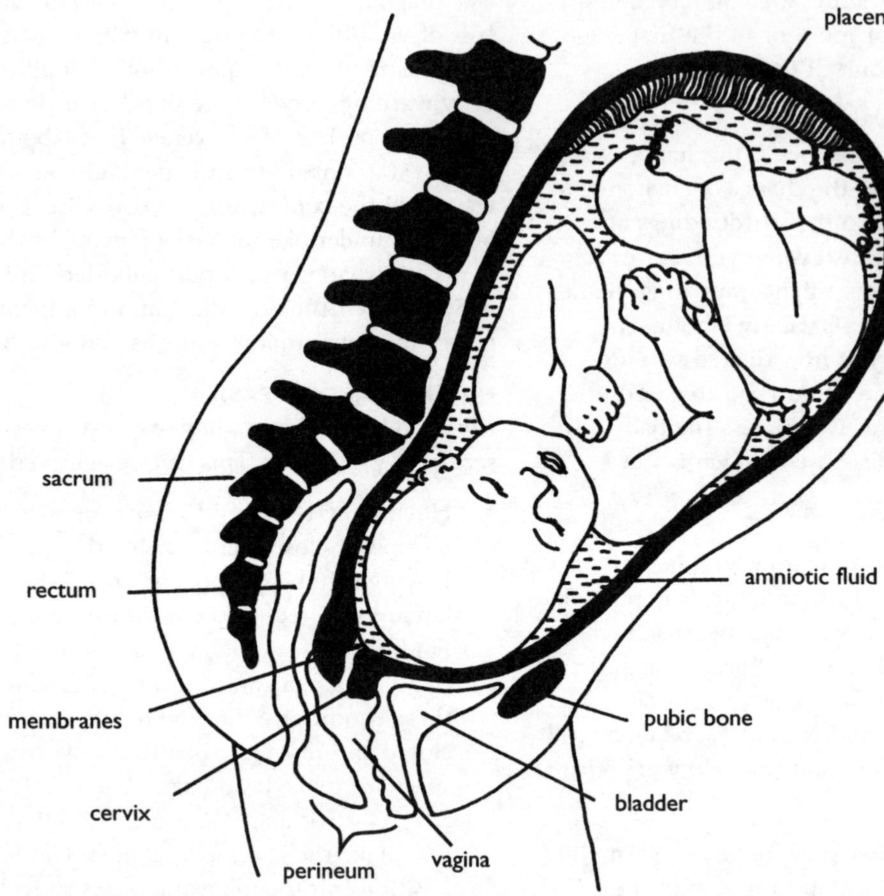

FIRST STAGE

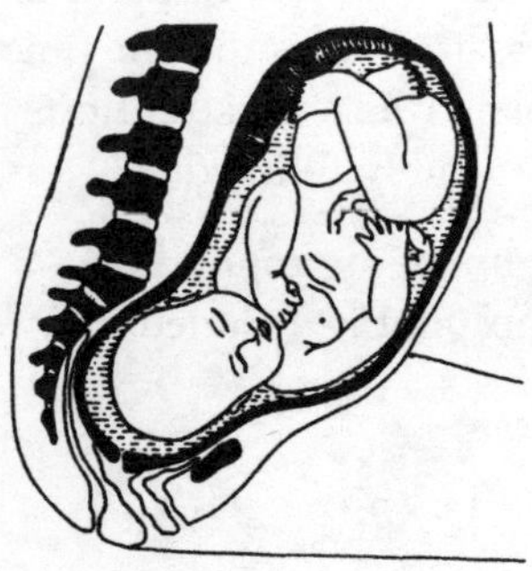

During this stage the cervix dilates from closed to open (0–10 cms). The baby moves down deeper into the pelvis, and the face gradually turns towards the mother's back.

Helping yourself

If you think that labour might be about to start:

- Conserve your energy, but keep on with your usual activities if it is daytime. If labour begins at night, try to rest, or sleep.
- Take a shower, go for a walk, but don't get tired.
- Don't skip any meals, particularly if labour starts during the night or early in the morning. Have something light, nourishing and easily digested such as scrambled eggs, tea and toast, soup.
- Pack the car with the things you wish to take to hospital, and also your labour 'goody bag'.
- Carry on with your usual daily routine until contractions become well established and you can be sure that labour really has begun.
- Contact your support people to alert them that you labour may be starting soon.

If the waters break note the colour of the fluid. It should be clear or milky white. If it is yellow/brown/green, then you should go to a hospital immediately, as this is a sign of possible fetal distress. See Preparing For Birth: Fathers.

If you begin labour before 37 weeks you should go to the hospital straight away as the baby may be born prematurely.

EARLY LABOUR

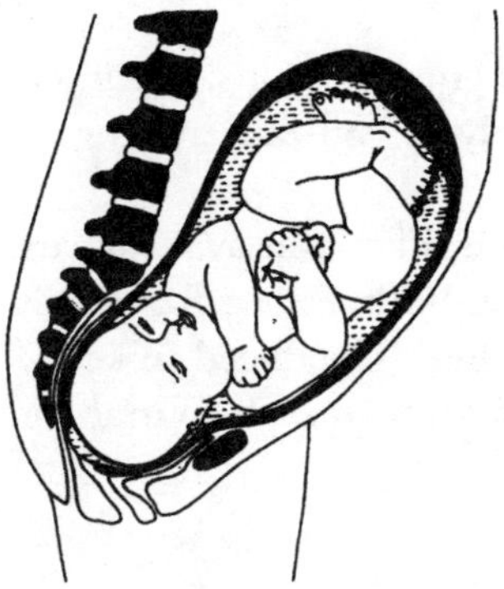

During this part of labour the cervix softens, shortens (effaces) and begins to dilate.

Helping yourself

- Continue eating as long as you feel like it.
- Have regular drinks of juice or water, about 1 cupful every hour.
- Move around until you find a comfortable position.
- Stay relaxed and avoid fatigue, but continue light activities as long as you feel able.
- Take each contraction as it comes, deal with it, then rest up for the next one. Listen to your body and find ways of making its work easier and more comfortable.
- Empty your bladder every 1–2 hours during labour.

ACCELERATED PHASE

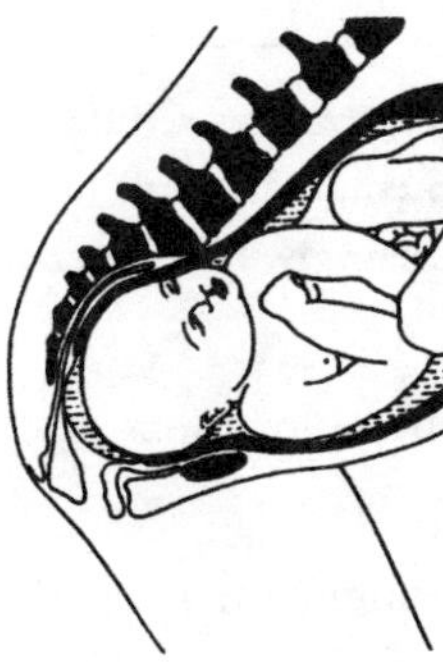

As dilatation reaches 4–5 cm labour enters the accelerated phase. Contractions will be stronger, closer together and will require concentration. You will feel the need to rest more between contractions. You will feel more introverted and focused on the activity within your body.

Helping yourself

- Conserve energy by finding positions where you can relax, fully supported, both during and between contractions.
- Keep drinking fluids, or if feeling nauseous, have sips of water or suck on ice chips. See Preparing For Birth: Fathers for more ideas.
- Have your support people provide massage or back rubs whenever you need them.
- In between contractions, ask support people for general massage, hot or cold packs or anything else you need to stay comfortable and relaxed. If your feet are cold, put on your woolly socks. See Preparing For Birth: Fathers for more ideas on dealing with the pain.
- If you are offered medication, request an internal examination to determine progress, before making a decision.
- A shower or bath at this time will help you to stay relaxed. Keep changing positions until you are comfortable.

TRANSITION

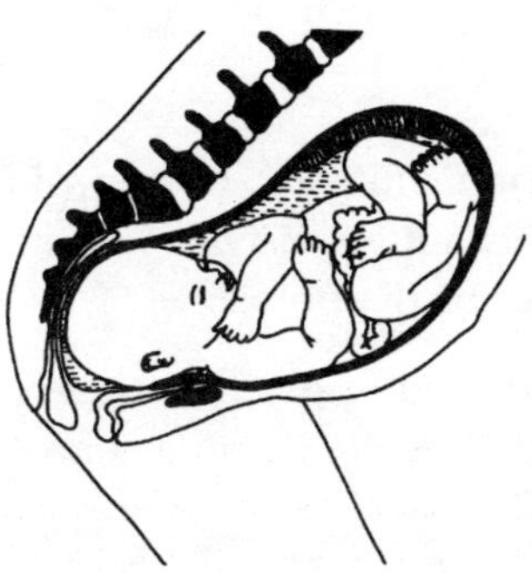

Transition is normally the most difficult part of labour, as your body is changing over from the opening up phase to the bearing down phase and contractions are usually very long (sometimes with double peaks) and close together.

It is a time of turbulent emotional feelings, and is often announced by sudden emotional change and feelings of being 'out of control'.

If the membranes haven't ruptured earlier this will probably happen during transition, and the release of pressure may ease some of the discomfort.

There may be an urge to push before the cervix is fully dilated. If pushing hurts at this time, then you should assume the knee-chest position until the cervix is fully retracted.

Other symptoms of transition are shivering, cramps, nausea, vomiting, hiccups. You may feel pressure on your bowel as the baby's head moves deeper into the birth canal. Transition usually lasts from a few contractions to around 1½ hours.

Helping yourself

This is a very turbulent time for most women, and feelings of panic, loss of control and annoying physical side-effects are all common. The support of your partner will be

TRANSITION (continued)

vital at this time, and suggestions on how he can help you are included in Preparing For Birth: Fathers.

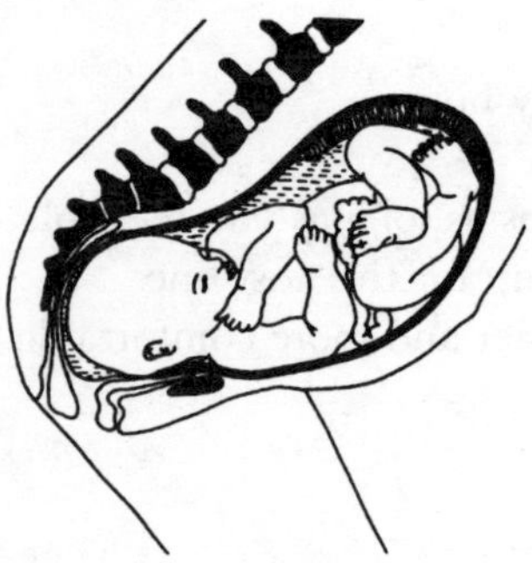

- You will have difficulty getting comfortable, but keep changing positions. It will be hard to stay relaxed, but concentrate on breathing as deeply as you can, making some noise with each out-breath to release the tension.
- A shower or bath at this time will give great pain relief, but if this is not available, use your hot, wet towels to provide local relief. See Preparing For Birth: Fathers for details.
- Support people need to hold, cuddle and reassure at this time. They need to keep distractions to a minimum, and concentrate on helping you through each contraction as it comes.
- Ice chips or sips of water will help dry lips and nausea.
- Cool sponges on face and neck feel good.
- Avoid eye contact and keep your eyes closed to avoid distractions.
- If the urge to push is felt prematurely, before dilatation is complete, move into the knee-chest position. Have pillows ready to lift your shoulders in between contractions.
- Reassurance and love are what you need most at this time.

SECOND STAGE

The second stage begins when the urge to push is felt. Sometimes there may be a lull between the end of the first stage and the first feelings of needing to push. If this lull occurs, take the opportunity for a rest until contractions re-establish strongly. This break from contractions may last up to 30 minutes or more.

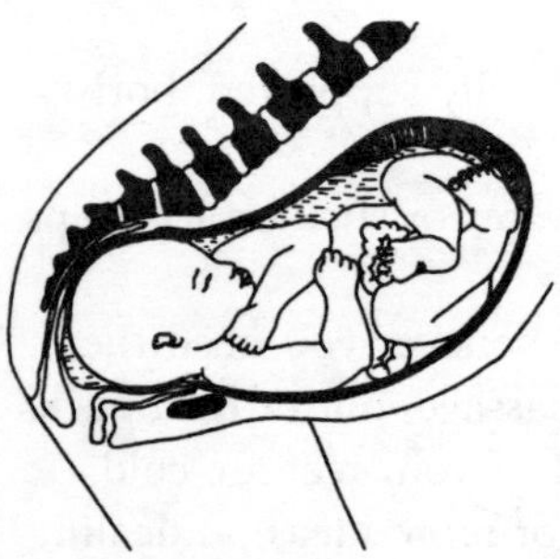

Contractions in second stage are usually shorter than in transition, and more spaced apart, with time to rest in between.

Second stage can last up to 2 or more hours with a first birth. Subsequent births are much shorter and stronger, usually about 1/2 hour for second stage.

The urge to bear down is usually irresistible. With each pushing action, the baby moves down the birth canal. Pressure will be felt on the bowel as the head presses on the rectum.

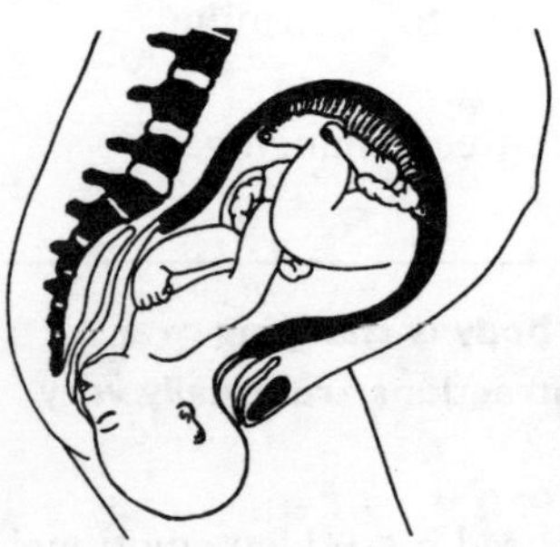

As the head presses on the perineum and the vaginal tissues open out, a burning sensation will develop as the skin stretches to its maximum. This is a signal to push gently as the baby's head crowns, to allow a gradual stretching and easing of the skin over the baby's face.

Once the head is born, it turns to one side to line up with the shoulders. The shoulders are born one at a time, and the baby's body slips out.

Helping yourself

Once the second stage begins the turbulent feelings of transition will pass and you will notice renewed energy: your second wind. Pushing usually feels quite satisfying as you work with your body and excitement is high as the moment of birth approaches.

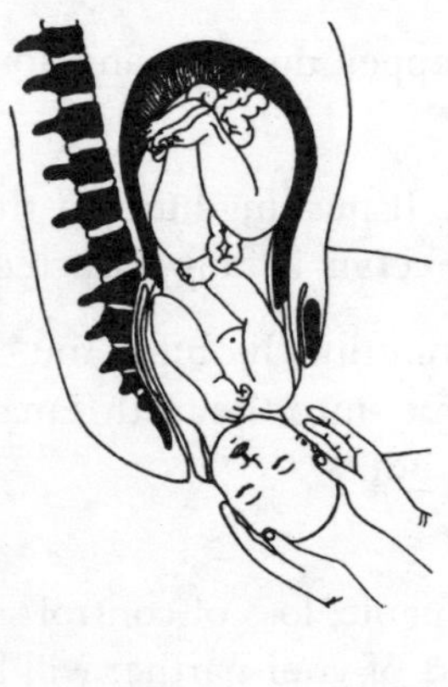

- The uterus will dictate when and how much to push – you need to listen to these messages from within and concentrate on letting your body open up. Find a comfortable position for pushing with your body upright and the sacrum free to move. In between contractions you can stand, kneel or flop forwards on to hands and knees.
- As you feel the burning sensation developing (crowning) concentrate on easing the baby out slowly. The burning sensation lasts less than a minute and will soon pass.
- Put your hand down to feel the top of the baby's head emerging from your vagina. In between contractions rest completely and keep sipping water.

THIRD STAGE OF LABOUR

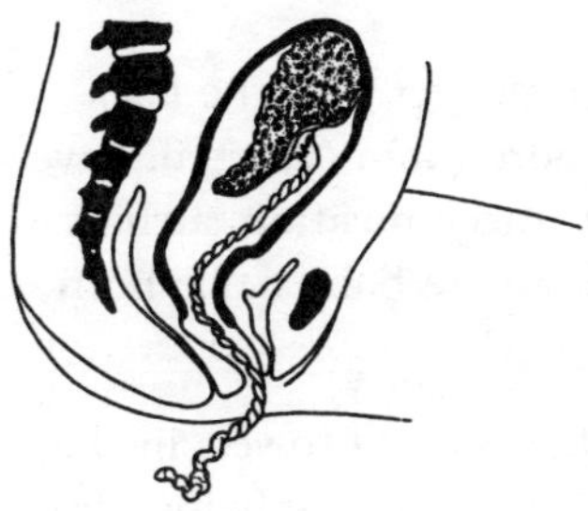

Once the baby is born, the cord usually stops pulsating within a few minutes. It can be clamped and cut either then or after the placenta has been born.

Meanwhile the uterus shrinks in size and continues to contract, a process helped by the baby nuzzling or sucking at the breast. The placenta begins to peel off the uterine wall and when free, slides into the vagina. Very gentle pulling on the cord will help it out, together with some pushes by the mother. The placenta is usually delivered after about 20 minutes. The placenta and membranes are examined to make sure they are complete and that no pieces have been trapped in the uterus.

The perineum is inspected to check for any grazes or tears that may need a stitch. If an episiotomy has been performed, then this will be repaired.

The baby is given to the mother to hold and the family left together to get to know their new baby.

During the first hour the baby will usually show signs of wanting to nurse at the breast. Encouraging the baby to suckle will help establish lactation and the sucking reflex in the baby, as well as helping the uterus to stay firmly contracted (important for preventing excessive bleeding).

Helping yourself

- Sit up while you are waiting for the placenta to come. This will help you see and hold the baby and facilitate latching on to the nipple. Skin-to-skin contact between you and the baby will help keep the baby warm, provide nipple stimulation and enhance the closeness.
- If you require stiches you will be offered a local anaesthetic (if you have not already received this in preparation for an episiotomy). You may find using the mask helps to relieve the pain of the anaesthetic injection.

Emergency birth

What should you do if the baby arrives before you reach hospital, or before your midwife arrives?

EMERGENCY BIRTH AT HOME

A very small proportion of women have a totally painless first stage of labour or experience mild contractions, and are unaware that anything is happening until they feel the urge to push, which is likely to be interpreted as a need to empty the bowel. Usually the waters will break at this time, which will alert you to the fact that this is the baby arriving.

Don't panic! This baby is going to arrive at home. If you do happen to be alone, phone your partner and anyone else who is to be with you, summon a neighbour or phone for an ambulance.

Go to a convenient place that is warm and quiet – the bathroom is ideal. Get into a comfortable position, with towels beneath you, and allow the baby to be born as slowly as possible – breathe the baby out.

Wipe any mucous from the baby's nose and mouth. The baby will probably cry straight away, but if not, lie the baby on its side on the towels, and massage the body firmly towards the head. Flicking the soles of the feet may also stimulate a cry.

It is important to keep the baby warm – wrap in a towel straight away and wait for the placenta. Put the baby to the breast if possible.

There is no need to cut the cord. When the placenta arrives, wrap it in a plastic bag and place it with the baby.

Phone the hospital and tell the midwife what has happened. When you are ready, make your way to the hospital, where the baby's cord will be cut and any tears will be repaired.

GIVING BIRTH ON THE WAY TO HOSPITAL

It is possible for the first stage of labour to progress so rapidly that you are ready to give birth in the car, before reaching hospital.

Again, don't panic! If there is time, get into the back seat of the car where there is more room (you will have to remove your pants) and get into a position such as hands and knees which will allow the baby to be born as slowly as possible.

It is useful to keep a couple of clean, old towels in the car to catch the fluids and for wrapping the baby. Make sure that the baby is breathing and pink and wrap up as warmly as possible before proceeding to hospital.

There is no need to cut the cord, and if the placenta does come appear, wrap it up and keep it with the baby.

CORD AROUND THE BABY'S NECK

It is very rare for the cord to be so tight that it stops the baby from being born. However, if the baby is not born with the next contraction after the head is out, feel round the baby's neck to see if there is a loop of cord. A loose loop can be gently eased over the head – there may even be two loops. If very tightly around the neck, the cord may have to be cut to allow the birth to proceed.

Tie two lengths of sewing tape/wide shoe laces (nothing very narrow) tightly around the cord, and with clean scissors (dip in Dettol/methylated spirit, wipe with soapy water if possible), cut in between the two ties. Unwrap the cord from round the neck. The rest of the baby can now be born. Make sure there is no bleeding from the cut ends.

Because this rare emergency could arise, it is suggested that an emergency pack, consisting of two clean lengths of tape and a pair of scissors be kept, wrapped in a clean plastic bag, in the bedroom. It should be put in the car when going to the hospital.

Comfort during labour and birth

There are many ways of increasing your comfort during labour. Making preparations in advance will increase your confidence in being able to help yourself and enable you to take care of your own needs without having to rely on the hospital staff. Being well-equipped and knowledgeable about self-help strategies will also reduce your need for pain killing drugs.

YOUR 'GOODY BAG'

Here are some suggestions for items to include in your 'goody bag'. All have proven useful for women in labour. Consider each one, and make your own list. Add any extras of your own.

Ways they can be used are described in Preparing For Birth: Fathers.

- An old T–shirt or loose top to wear
- Several pairs of panties and some sanitary pads – to catch leaking fluid
- Dressing gown and slippers – for walking around the labour ward
- Your own pillow(s)
- The duvet from your bed
- Aromatherapy oil burner (electric) – for creating a relaxing environment
- Shower hat – to keep hair dry under the shower
- Fruit juice – to drink every hour during labour
- Glucose lollies to suck – for extra energy
- Vegetable oil – for massage (aromatherapy oils such as lavender are a nice addition)
- Face cloth – for wiping sweaty foreheads
- Warm socks – feet get very cold in labour!
- Lip chapstick – for dry lips
- 4 hand towels, rubber gloves and bucket – to make hot towels for relief of pain anywhere.
- The gloves should be large enough for the support person to wear. Use the bucket to carry everything on your 'goody bag' list.
- Tennis balls – provide firm local pressure
- Food and drinks – for your support people to keep their energy up
- Swim suit or change of clothes for your support person – for use in the shower
- Tape recorder, earphones and music tapes – to help you relax
- Camera – to record the event. Use 1000 ASA film and you won't need a flash
- This book and Preparing For Birth: Fathers – to remind you of positions for labour and helpful ideas for any problems.

MY 'GOODY BAG' LIST:

Positions for labour – First stage

On the following pages are some suggestions for positions you may find useful during labour. Experiment with these in pregnancy to find those that seem most comfortable, but be prepared to try them all again when labour is underway. In choosing the most comfortable position, remember:

- The woman should be as fully supported as possible, using people, pillows, bean bags or furniture, to allow her to fully relax.
- Knees should be bent to avoid tiredness in the legs and to make pelvic rocking easier.
- Her feet should be apart to give a wide base for support, and to encourage 'open' positions.
- Be creative in your adaptation of available furniture in the hospital. If you need extra pillows or a stool or chair, request these.
- Once a comfortable position is found, use it until she signals that it is no longer helping her relax. Change positions only as she indicates, unless you are positioning for a specific purpose, such as to help the baby turn from posterior or to encourage the baby to move down further into the pelvis.

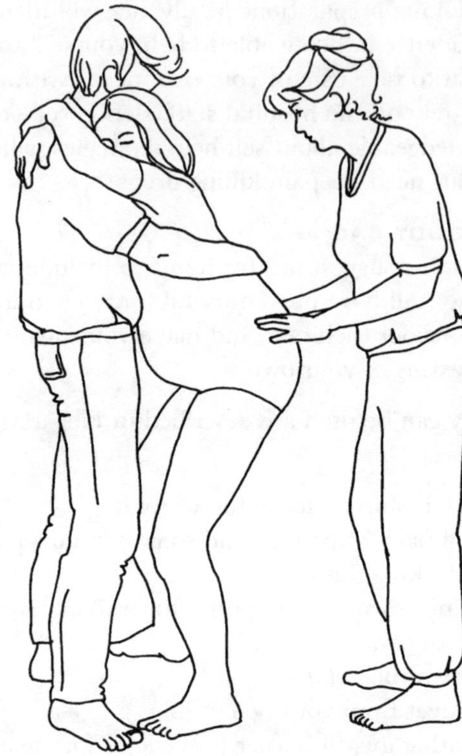

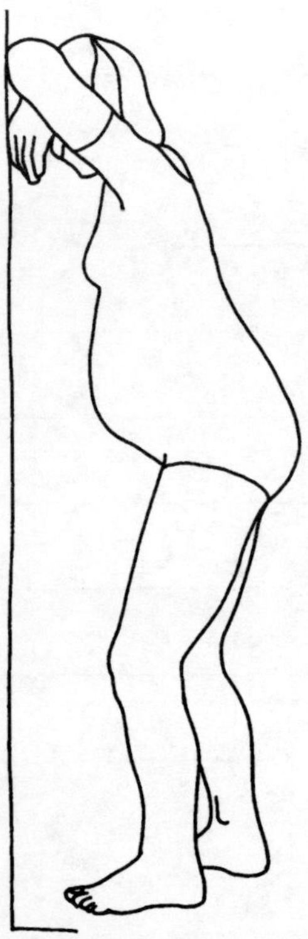

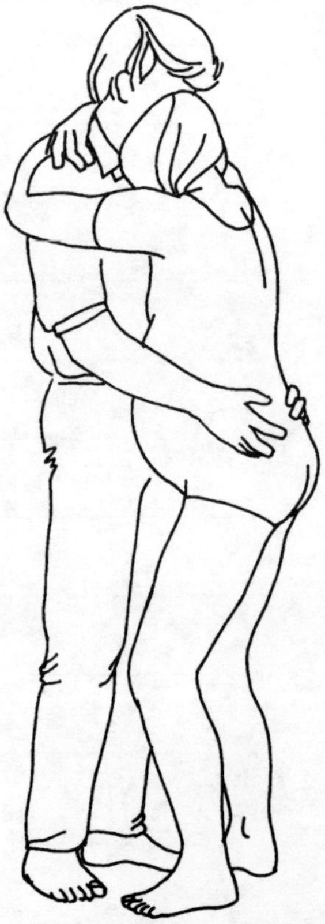

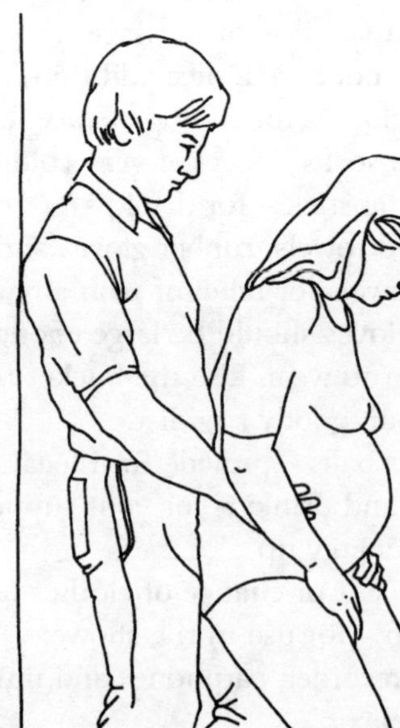

Positions for labour – First stage

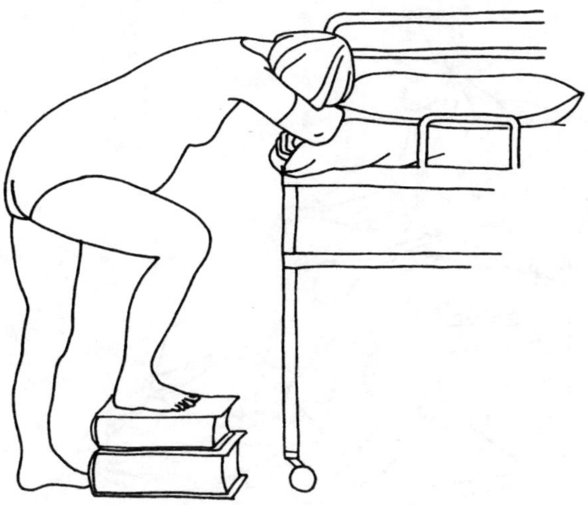

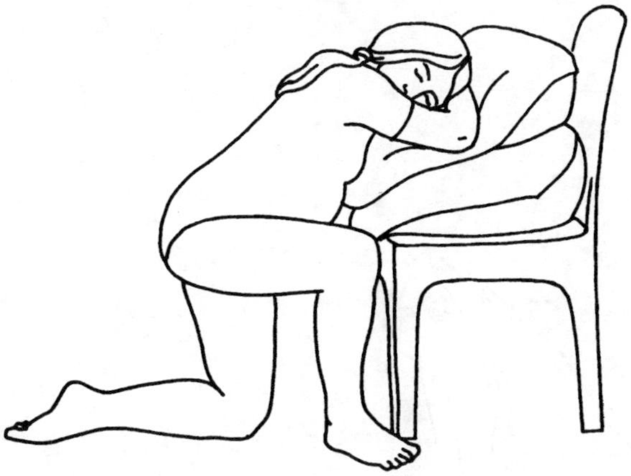

Some women find asymmetrical positions help ease pressure points.

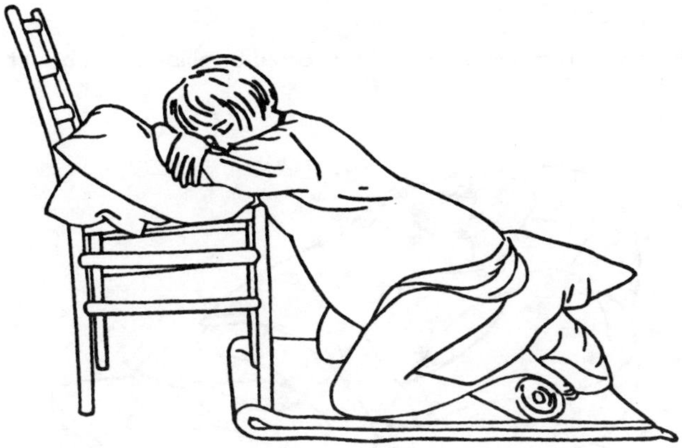

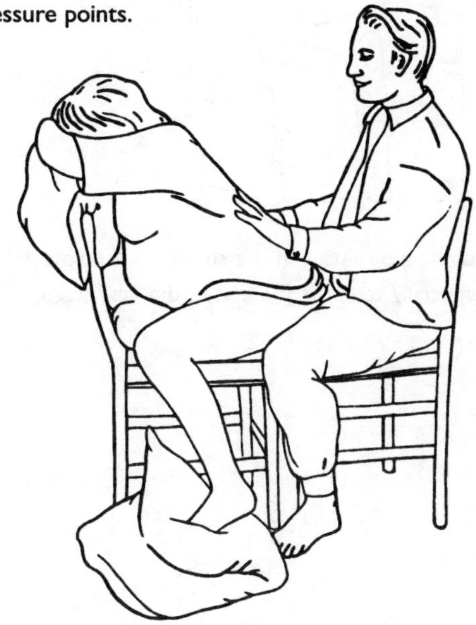

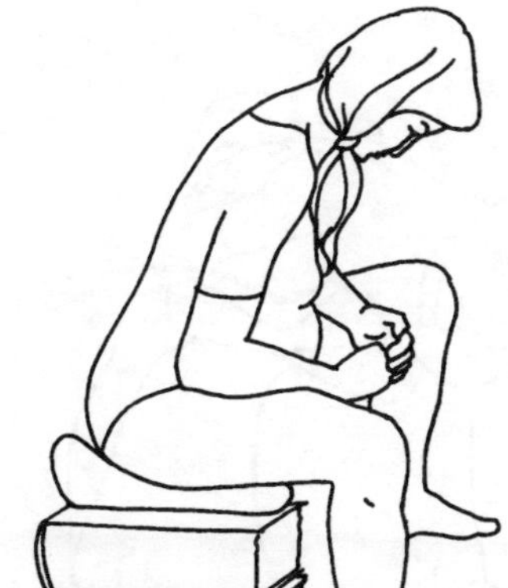

You can easily use a bedpan like this.

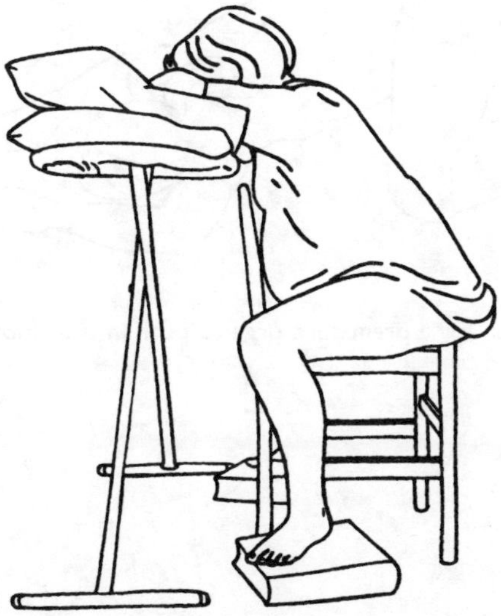

Positions for labour – Transition

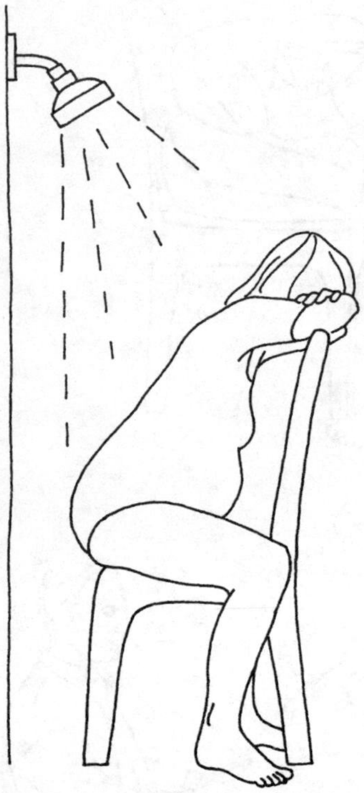

Standing or sitting in the shower will help ease much of the pain, especially towards the end of the first stage.

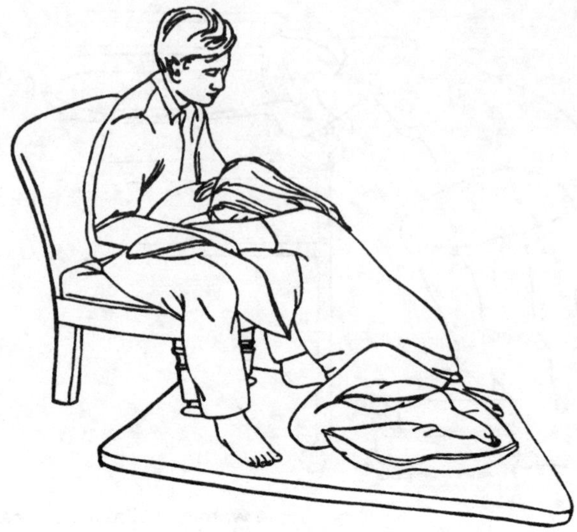

It is easy to rest if you are well supported by pillows or a bean bag.

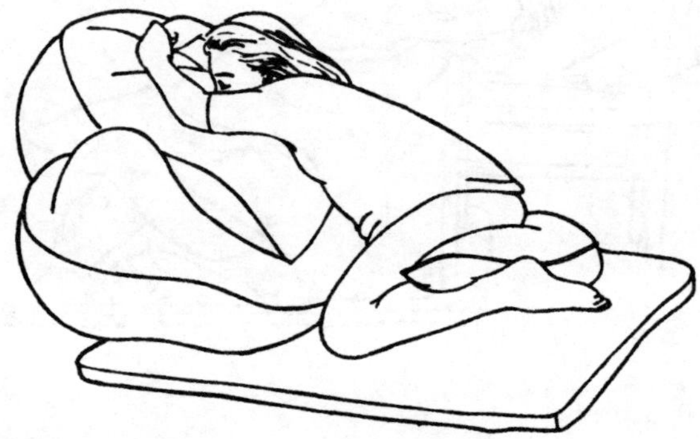

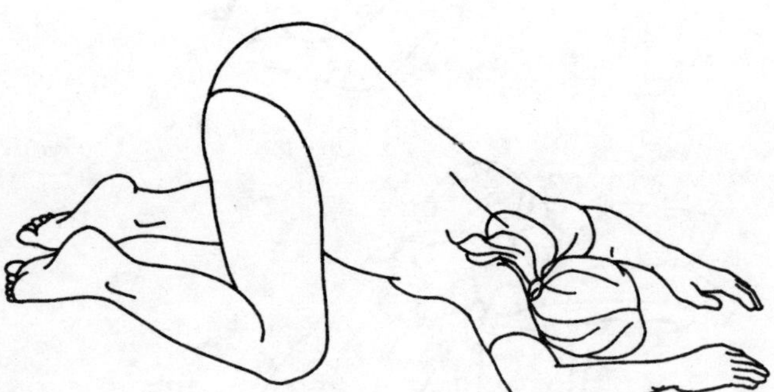

Knee-chest position for a premature urge to push in transition.

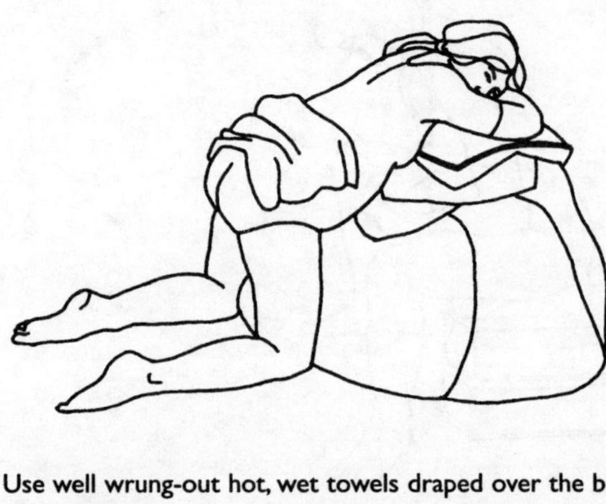

Use well wrung-out hot, wet towels draped over the buttocks for lower back pain.

Positions for labour – Second stage

In second stage, a woman needs to be able to brace her body to push effectively. She will seek something to grip and will prefer to be upright with her feet planted firmly on a floor mat and good support from her partner or other helpers. Furniture can also be used as a source of support.

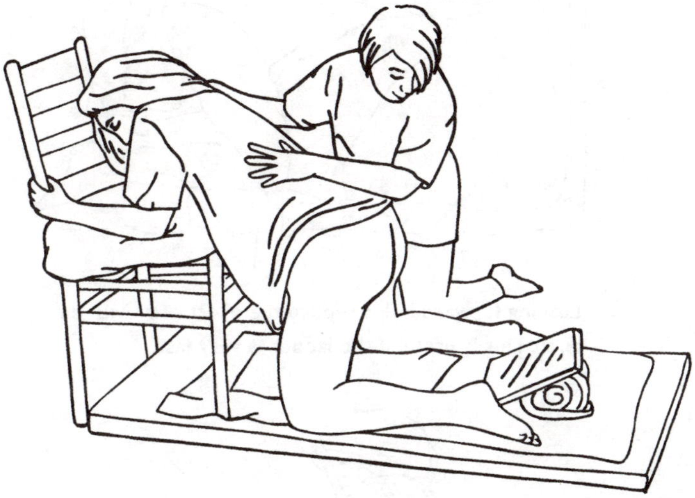

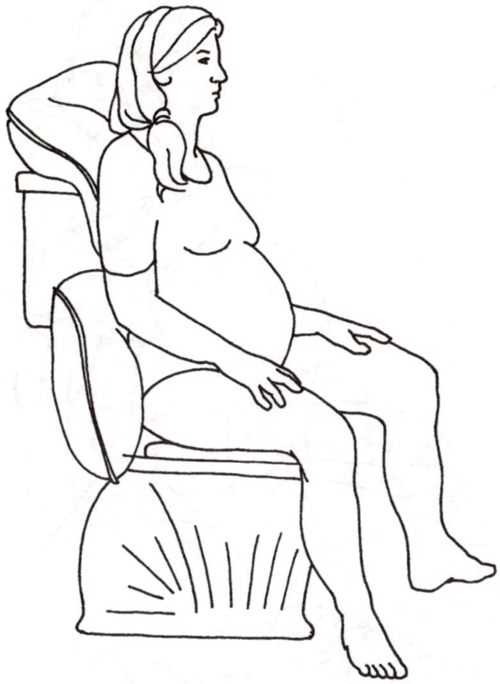

Sitting on the toilet often helps early pushing contractions become more coordinated.

A mirror is useful to enable the father and caregivers to see the baby's progress towards birth. Women usually have their eyes tightly closed at this time!

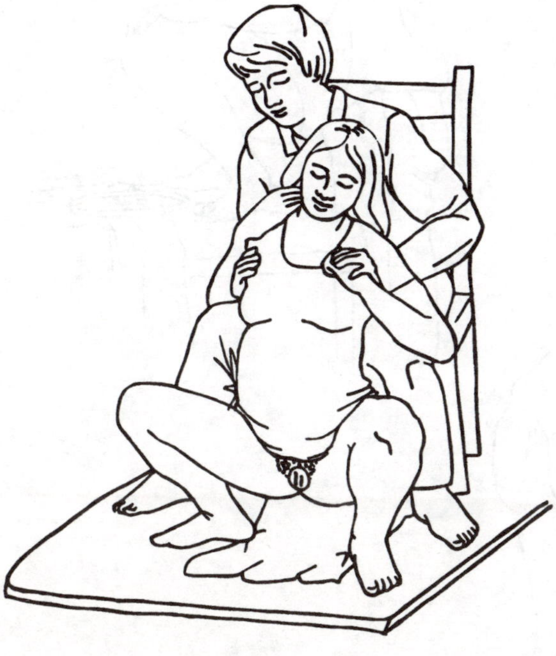

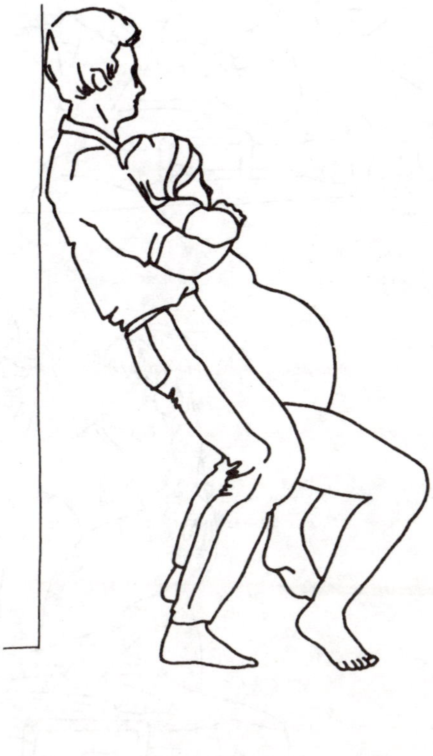

Positions for labour – Second stage

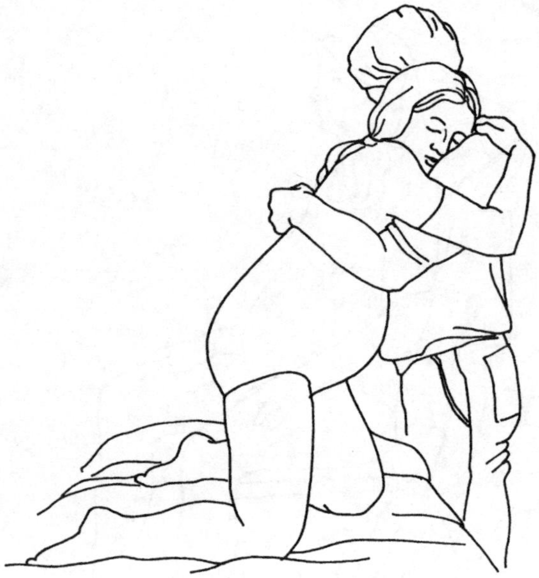

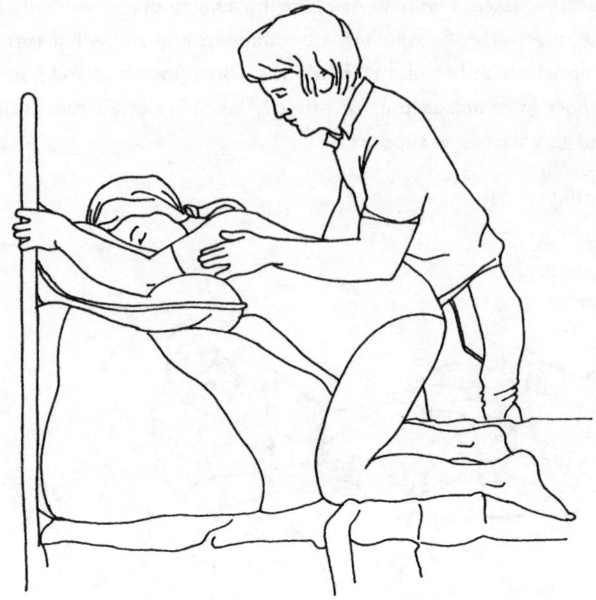

Leaning forward helps reduce the effect of gravity during birth. This is useful if the labour is very fast.

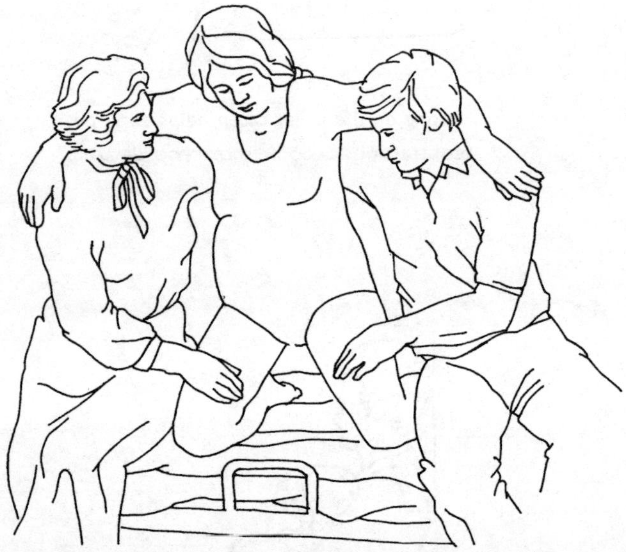

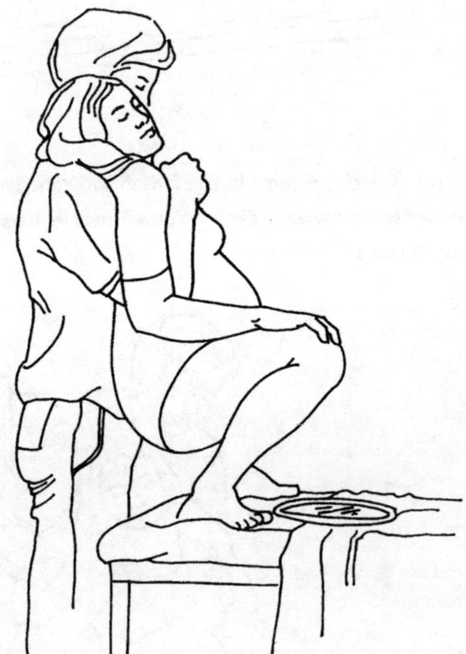

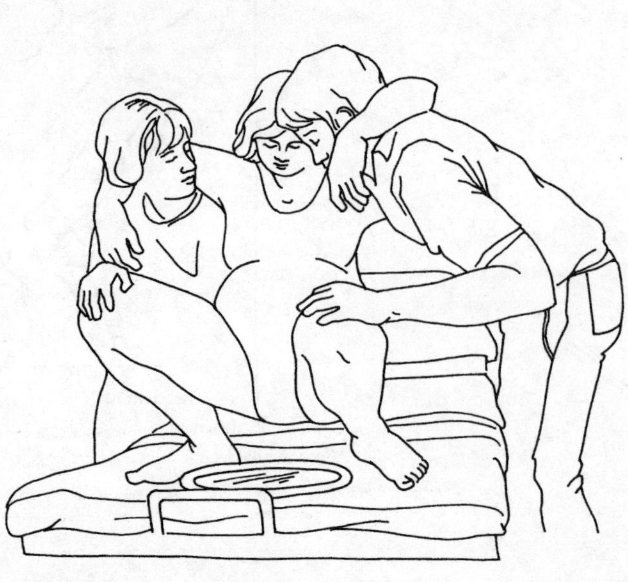

Obstetric interventions explained

Obstetric interventions can be life-saving procedures for women and babies. Technological advances, improved surgical techniques and better anaesthetics have ensured that the 20% of women who need this kind of help receive the best possible care.

Once the natural process of labour and birth has been disturbed, especially if there is no actual medical emergency, there is a significant risk that the unwelcome side effects of the treatment will make further intervention necessary to remedy the problem.

This phenomenon is known as 'the cascade of intervention' and is illustrated in the diagram.

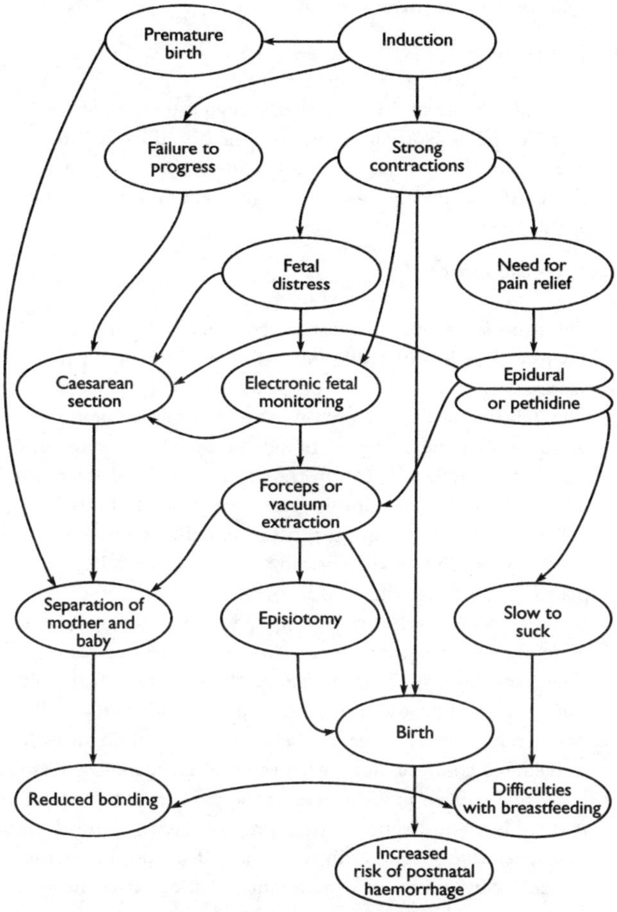

All the links shown have been proven by scientific research.
To read the diagram, start with the intervention being considered and read downwards from that point.

THE USE OF ARTIFICIAL OXYTOCICS IN LABOUR

The body produces a natural hormone, oxytocin, which makes the uterus contract during labour. Synthetic oxytocin (Syntocinon) can be given to a mother for three main reasons:

- To start labour artificially (induction). In this case the procedure often involves rupturing the membranes (see separate entry).
- To speed up labour (augmentation) after labour starts naturally, or if labour slows down, perhaps in response to other interventions (e.g. epidural administration).
- To speed up the delivery of the placenta (active management of third stage) and to control post-partum bleeding.

Each of these possibilities will be considered in turn.

INDUCTION USING AN OXYTOCIN DRIP

When is it necessary?

- If the mother's health or life would be endangered by continuing the pregnancy, for example:
  - severe pre-eclampsia (also known as toxaemia or pregnancy induced hypertension)
  - kidney disease
  - heart condition
  - diabetes
- If the baby's health or well-being is being compromised by remaining in the uterus. For example:
  - signs of placental dysfunction, when the baby is not being properly fed by the placenta
  - membranes ruptured for more than 48 hours with no contractions, and signs of developing infection.
- Less clear-cut reasons, such as:
  - being overdue
  - social reasons
  - doctor's or mother's convenience.

How is it done?

A drip line is attached to a vein in the back of the hand, and synthetic oxytocin (Syntocinon) is steadily released into the body via the drip. The drip is attached to a device which monitors the rate of flow and this rate is gradually increased until contractions are established, lasting one minute and coming every two minutes.

Effects on the mother

Advantages:

- A usually reliable method of bringing on the labour when life or health is at risk.
- Social reasons: being able to organise the birth when help is available for other children or the partner can be present.

Disadvantages:

- A more painful and stressful labour should be anticipated.
- Increased need for analgesic drugs, for example pethidine, epidurals.
- Unless the cervix is ready to dilate, the progress will be slow and may lead to a Caesarean section for 'failure to progress'.
- If the mother is immobilised in bed she will be less able to find comfortable positions for labour. It should be possible to provide a mobile drip stand; however the attachment of the drip into the back of the hand is often inconvenient.
- If an epidural is needed, or exhaustion results from a long, painful labour there is an increased risk of forceps delivery.
- Greater chance of early separation of mother and baby due to adverse effects of drugs used or routine following an assisted delivery.
- Over-riding of the body's natural production of oxytocin causes decreased sensitivity to naturally released oxytocin in response to the suckling of the baby at the breast. This can lead to difficulty establishing lactation in the first few days post-partum.

Effects on the baby

Advantages:

- A usually reliable means of bringing on the labour when the baby's health may be at risk.
- The baby can be born at a time when specialist attention and facilities are available, for example, paediatrician for 'at-risk' babies.

Disadvantages:

- The strength and length of contractions may cause fetal distress due to lack of oxygen, and necessitate further intervention.

- Increased likelihood of jaundice developing caused by the presence of drugs, (e.g. Syntocinon, pethidine) in the baby's system after birth which have to be metabolised and eliminated at the same time as the extra red blood cells all babies have after birth.
- An assisted birth and/or large amounts of analgesia, especially pethidine, may cause baby to have breathing difficulties and a weak sucking reflex.
- Early separation of mother and baby if any of these problems are severe.
- Increased risk of prematurity if the baby's birth is before term.

AUGMENTATION OF LABOUR

When is it necessary?

- If the labour slows down and there is evidence that the prolonged labour is jeopardising the baby's well-being.
- If the labour slows down as a side effect of epidural anaesthesia, artificial oxytocin must be given to help re-establish the contractions.

How is it done?

A drip is set up in the same way as for an induction, but after labour has started naturally. If labour slows down following an epidural, then Syntocinon is given to the mother via the drip that has been set up as part of the epidural procedure.

Effects on the mother

Advantages:

- Makes labour shorter and may reduce maternal exhaustion from a long labour.

Disadvantages:

- The labour may be more painful and stressful due to unnaturally long contractions coming at frequent intervals, giving little time to rest.
- Increased need for pain relieving drugs, for example pethidine or an epidural. Having an epidural may slow labour, resulting in the need for increased levels of Syntocinon.
- Over-riding the body's natural levels of oxytocin will decrease sensitivity to natural oxytocin production post-partum and could pose problems in establishing lactation.

Effects on the baby

Advantages:

- The baby will be born sooner.

Disadvantages:

- The increased intensity of contractions may cause fetal distress due to reduced oxygen supply during long contractions with little recovery time between. This may necessitate further interventions, such as forceps or Caesarean, if the problem is severe.
- Increased likelihood of jaundice developing caused by the presence of drugs, (e.g. Syntocinon, pethidine) in the baby's system after birth which have to be metabolised and eliminated at the same time as the extra red blood cells all babies have after birth
- An assisted birth and/or large amounts of analgesic drugs may interfere with the baby's breathing at birth and cause weak sucking reflexes.
- Early separation of mother and baby if any of these problems are severe.

ACTIVE MANAGEMENT OF THIRD STAGE

An injection of Syntocinon (or sometimes Syntometrine, a mixture of oxytocin and ergometrine) is given to the mother as the baby is being born to speed up the separation of the placenta and hasten its arrival. The injection is also given to reduce the chance of haemorrhage after the birth.

When is it necessary?

- Poor obstetric history (for example previous post-partum haemorrhage, incoordinate uterine contractions).
- Low haemoglobin levels in the blood (anaemia) which could mean delay in blood clotting.
- Following a Caesarean section.

How is it done?

- The Syntocinon (or Syntometrine) can be given either by injection usually into the mother's thigh after the baby is born, or if a drip line is in place, through the drip directly into a vein.
- The cord is clamped and cut immediately after the baby is born.
- The cord is pulled to encourage early separation and delivery of the placenta.

Effects on the mother

Advantages:

- The third stage of labour can be completed rapidly.
- There will be less bleeding immediately after the birth.

Disadvantages:

- The delivery of the placenta must be completed before the uterus, under the influence of large amounts of oxytocin, contracts sufficiently to trap the placenta behind the closing cervix. Once the injection is given, the placenta must be delivered within 10 minutes to prevent this happening.
- Excessive pulling on the cord in an attempt to deliver the placenta can cause the cord to break.
- If the placenta does become trapped in the uterus, then a manual removal under general anaesthetic will be needed. The doctor uses his hand to scrape the placenta off the uterine wall and bring it out through the vagina. This will usually be done under a spinal or general anaesthetic but if no anaesthetist is available could be done with the mother using the nitrous oxide and oxygen mask to relieve the pain from the procedure.
- If there is an undiagnosed twin present, giving Syntocinon may cause the second twin to be caught inside the uterus. A Caesarean section or general anaesthetic may be needed to deliver the baby.
- High levels of artificial oxytocin may cause reduced sensitivity to natural levels of oxytocin released in response to sucking by the baby, and lead to difficulties with the let-down reflex and establishment of lactation in the fist days post-partum.

PROSTAGLANDINS

A hormone, in gel form, applied to the cervix in preparation for an induction.

When is it necessary?

- To help soften the cervix prior to inducing labour before term.
- At term, to initiate labour without using a drip or rupturing the membranes.

How is it done?

- The prostaglandins is applied as a gel in the area around the cervix.
- A repeat dose may be used after 6 hours.
- Not recommended for women with ruptured membranes.

Effects on the mother

Advantages:

- May initiate a more physiologic labour than an induction by other means.

Disadvantages:

- May cause severe spontaneous labour if the cervix is already ripe.
- Increased risk of infection.
- Nausea, vomiting and diarrhoea may occur.
- Increased risk of post-partum haemorrhage.

Effect on baby

Advantages:

- May initiate a more physiologic and less stressful labour than induction by other means.

Disadvantages:

- Increased risk of fetal distress.

ARTIFICIAL RUPTURE OF THE MEMBRANES

This is the artificial breaking of the membranes surrounding the baby, releasing the amniotic fluid.

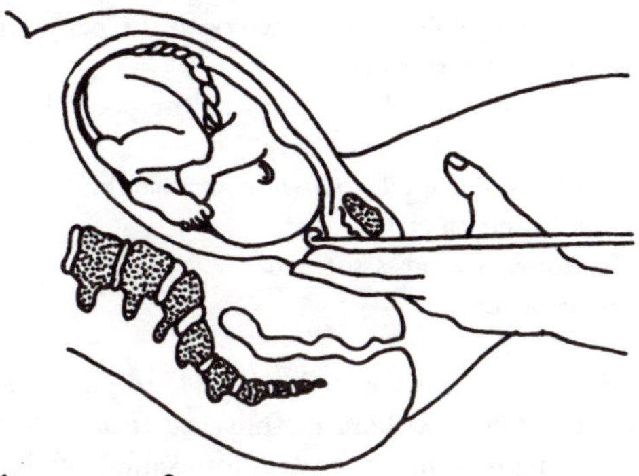

When is it necessary?

- To assist in the induction of labour (usually used in conjunction with oxytocic drugs).
- To speed up labour which has started naturally (augmentation).
- To check the colour of the amniotic fluid if fetal distress is suspected.

How is it done?

The mother is asked to lie on her back with legs open. A long plastic tube with a sharp hook on the end (similar to a crochet hook) is introduced through the vagina and cervix. A small nick is made in the membranes and the fluid is allowed to escape.

Effects on the mother

Advantages:

- Research has shown that labour may be shortened by an average of up to one hour.

Disadvantages:

- As the cushion of fluid between the baby's head and the cervix is removed, the fetal head presses firmly on the cervix. This has the effect of causing very strong contractions, due to direct pressure on the cervix by the hard head.
- The increased intensity of the contractions may cause rapid dilatation and extra pain and discomfort. If early in labour, the intense contractions may lead to an increased use of pain-relieving drugs. If late in labour, then the mother may be suddenly thrown into transition without warning
- With the membranes ruptured, there is an increased risk of infection. Time limits may be placed on the length of labour from that point to avoid further complications.
- Once the fluid is reduced there is an increased risk of compression of the umbilical cord, which may reduce the flow of blood and oxygen to the baby from the placenta.

Effects on the baby

Advantages:

- The labour may be shorter.

Disadvantages:

- The extra pressure on the fetal head may cause distress to the baby, and lead to further interventions to assist the baby.
- The pain-relieving drugs required by the mother have side-effects on the baby.
- Prolonged rupture of membranes may lead to infection in the baby.

ELECTRONIC FETAL MONITORING

An electronic method of determining the baby's heart rate, the strength and length of contractions and the reaction of the baby to those contractions.

When is it necessary?

- When there are signs of fetal distress indicating that the baby may be experiencing difficulties during the labour.
- When an epidural has removed the mother's ability to interpret the strength and timing of her contractions.
- Commonly used when labour is being induced to determine the effects of the induction on the baby.

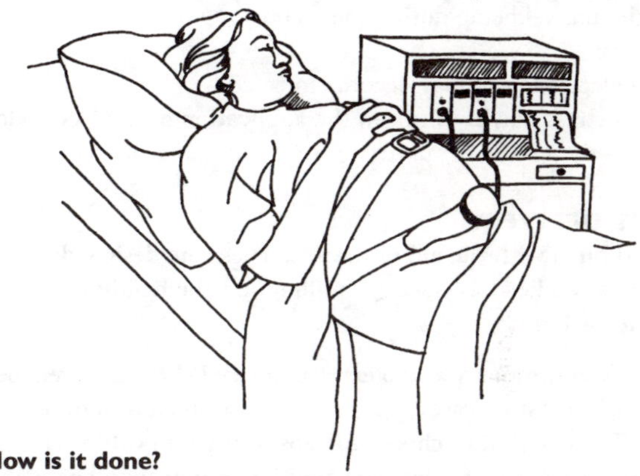

How is it done?

External monitoring uses two large elastic belts positioned around the abdomen. One holds a transducer (in a plastic disc) which emits an ultrasound beam to record the baby's heartbeat, the other belt records the strength and length of the contractions using a similar transducer. The belts are wired up to a machine that provides a printout of both readings. Internal monitoring provides the same information, but via an electrode attached to the baby's scalp (heart rate) and a fine tube inside the uterine cavity (contractions). Sometimes an external belt instead of an internal tube is used to measure the contractions. Rupture of the membranes is necessary to attach the scalp electrode.

Effects on the mother

Advantages:

- Can be reassuring to have constant feedback about the condition of the baby.
- Allows the mother to visually monitor the labour which she may be unable to feel if she has an epidural.

Disadvantages:

- The mother is often restricted to bed and must remain still for the monitor to record well. This restricts her choices of positions for labour.

- Transient variations in the baby's heartbeat may cause undue alarm and lead to further interventions which may later prove unjustified. Research shows that there is considerable disagreement on the interpretation of EFM printouts, even amongst experts viewing the same graph. This means there is likely to be both false positive and false negative results recorded.
- Because internal monitoring is more accurate, early rupture of the membranes may be performed to allow a scalp electrode to be inserted. This procedure itself may cause fetal distress from increased direct pressure of the fetal head on the cervix with longer and stronger contractions.
- The machine may become the focus of attention rather than the mother.
- The effects of the exposure of mother and baby to long periods of ultrasound from the transducers are unknown.
- Research has shown that electronic fetal monitoring is of no benefit in normal labours but significantly increases the chances of a Caesarean section or forceps delivery. The baby's heartbeat can be noted just as effectively using a fetal stethoscope, with no side effects.

Effects on the baby

Advantages:

- May enable early detection of potential risks to the baby's health and wellbeing during the labour.

Disadvantages:

- Scalp electrode site may become infected.
- Fetal distress may result from the application of the electrode or from the results of rupturing the membranes prematurely.

FORCEPS DELIVERY

An assisted birth with the aid of forceps. These are designed to cradle the baby's head as traction (pulling) on the handles assists the baby to be born.

Research has shown that vacuum extraction (see below) is preferable to forceps in almost all cases as it causes less trauma to mother and baby. The decision to choose forceps or vacuum will often depend on caregiver preference and training, rather than being based on scientific evidence.

When is it necessary?

Forceps are used only during second stage, and for these reasons:

- A delay in second stage, perhaps due to an unfavourable position of the baby. The forceps can be used to rotate the head so it can be more easily born.
- To enable the baby to be born if an epidural has left the mother with no urge to push especially if she is lying on her back.
- Fetal distress, when it is necessary to have the baby born quickly.
- To protect the head if the baby is premature or in the breech position.
- Maternal exhaustion or a condition where pushing would be detrimental to the mother, for example a maternal heart condition or a very high blood pressure.
- Sometimes forceps are used to lift the baby out if second stage is considered to be taking too long. If progress is slow then a change of positions (preferably to an open, upright position) should be tried before forceps are used to speed up the birth.

It should be noted that the use of analgesia, especially epidurals, leads to increased likelihood of a forceps birth. The anaesthetic numbs the pelvic floor muscles making it difficult for them to guide the baby's head into a favourable position for birth. Having to lie down for the birth also removes the effect of gravity and makes if difficult to push up hill, especially when the urge to push is severely diminished or absent and a forceps 'lift-out' is the likely outcome.

How is it done?

- The cervix must be fully dilated.
- The bladder should be empty – a catheter may be used to achieve this.
- The mother is placed in the lithotomy position (on her back with her legs supported in stirrups).
- Some form of local anaesthetic is administered, if an epidural is not already in place.
- The forceps blades are inserted one at a time and locked into position around the baby's head.
- If necessary the doctor rotates the head into a favourable position.
- The head is then pulled right down onto the perineum.
- An episiotomy is performed.
- The baby's head is lifted out and then the body. The baby is treated and observed as necessary.
- The placenta is delivered, following an injection of Syntocinon or ergometrine.
- The episiotomy wound is sutured.

Effects on the mother

Advantages:

- When the mother is exhausted or unable to push it allows the baby to be born without her physical effort.
- When pushing is contra-indicated, for example with severe pre-eclampsia, the baby can be born.

Disadvantages:

- Because the birth is assisted, the mother misses the experience of pushing the baby out herself.
- The local or epidural anaesthetic numbs the perineal area so that the mother doesn't feel the baby emerging.
- An episiotomy is usually routine.
- The need for analgesia, often a pudendal block, or an epidural.
- Bruising of internal tissues, and additional strain on pelvic floor muscles.

Effects on the baby

Advantages:

- Where fetal distress is present, a forceps delivery may be life-saving, or prevent the baby from becoming very hypoxic (oxygen-starved) which, if severe, can lead to brain damage or death.
- May be necessary to protect the baby's head, for example a premature birth or breech presentation.
- May be the only way that birth can be achieved, if the baby is malpositioned.

Disadvantages:

- In the hands of an experienced doctor there should be little trauma to the baby. There may be some bruising or temporary markings on the baby's face.
- The baby may suffer from the effects of the increased need for analgesia.
- There is always some degree of force used in a forceps delivery and it is difficult to know what effect this force has on the baby's head and spine. If your baby has been born with the

aid of forceps and is very irritable, it might be worthwhile having its neck checked for misalignment of the vertebrae in its spine.

VENTOUSE (VACUUM EXTRACTION)

This is an alternative to forceps, when the baby requires assistance to be born.

When is it necessary?

The indications for its use are similar to those for forceps, with some differences:

- Vacuum extraction can be performed before the cervix is completely open, as the suction cup takes no additional space around the baby's head. This may enable a very distressed baby to be born quickly. It is not usually used for premature or breech births. It is impossible to apply strong pressure to the baby's head with the vacuum device, as it will slip off if excessive force is used. The small size of the device reduces the risk of damage to the mother's vaginal tissues.

How is it done?

- The mother is placed in the lithotomy position (on her back) with her legs in stirrups.
- A suction cup is applied to the baby's head and held in place while the suction (generated from a portable suction pump or obtained through the hospital's in-built suction system) draws the skin on the scalp firmly into the cup.
- Handles attached to the vacuum extractor can then be used to turn the baby and gently lift it out.
- The mother must assist by pushing.
- Once the head is born, the suction cup is removed and the baby is born normally.
- The 'chignon' or lump on the baby's head caused by the suction usually disappears within hours.

Effects on the mother

Advantages:

- Can be used before the cervix is fully dilated if rapid delivery is indicated by the baby's condition.
- An episiotomy is not usually required.
- Very little, if any, internal bruising of the maternal tissues.
- Mother can still feel the birth and be involved by assisting with pushing.

Disadvantages:

- This technique is not always available, due to lack of experience or professional preferences.
- The technique may fail due to repeated inability of the suction cup to stay in place, and either forceps or a Caesarean may then be necessary.

Effects on the baby

Advantages:

- The baby can be born before the cervix is fully dilated, which could be helpful to a distressed infant in need of being born.
- Less likelihood of displacement of the neck bones as the forces applied by vacuum extraction are not as great as those with forceps.
- Fewer marks on the head and face. The marks left by the suction cap disappear very quickly.

Disadvantages:

- The 'chignon' lump on the baby's head will take time to disappear.
- The baby may be distressed by having suction applied to its head and by traction during the birth.

EPISIOTOMY

An cut (made with scissors) in the perineal tissues at the time of birth.

When is it necessary?

- To protect the premature baby's head from undue pressure during birth.
- To allow more space for the application of forceps.
- To protect the baby's head if the perineum is tight and unyielding or is delaying the birth of the baby.
- To speed up second stage.

How is it done?

The mother is asked to lie back so that a clear view of the perineum can be obtained.

- Local anaesthetic is injected in several places close to where the tissues will be cut.
- If the cut is made when the skin is numb from stretching, then no anaesthesia may be needed until stitching begins.
- When the head is crowning, the doctor or midwife makes a surgical cut, using scissors, from the base of the vagina either out to the side (lateral) or down towards the anus (midline). Occasionally a J-shaped incision is made, to the side.
- Dissolving stitches are used which disappear within 1–2 weeks.

Effects on the mother

Advantages:

- An episiotomy may speed up labour by removing the need to wait for tissues and skin to stretch during second stage.
- An episiotomy may be preferable to an uncontrolled tear if the birth is fast or the tissues are very tight.

Disadvantages:

- An episiotomy done before the perineal area has fully stretched will involve cutting much tissue and a significant blood loss as a consequence.
- Episiotomies frequently tear further, causing a bigger wound. If extensive, this tearing can involve the anus and make extensive surgical repair necessary. Involvement of the anal sphincter can lead to weakness and problems with incontinence.
- An episiotomy takes longer to heal and is more painful than a tear, as muscle tissue is involved in an episiotomy. Tears usually involve only skin and superficial tissue, and therefore heal faster.
- Healing can take months for some women. Sexual difficulties and general pain and discomfort may be felt until healing is complete. Further repair work may be necessary.
- Having a sore perineum and stitches that require care can interfere with the ability to take care of a baby in the first days post-partum.

Effects on the baby

Advantages:

- Shortens second stage
- Prevents undue pressure on the head of a premature baby.

Disadvantages:

- A sore and tender perineum can make it more difficult for the mother to care for the baby after the birth.

CAESAREAN SECTION

This is the delivery of the baby through a surgical incision made in the abdominal wall and the lowest part of the uterus.

When is it necessary?

- Pre-eclampsia (hypertensive disorder).
- Fetal distress.
- Failure to progress in labour – often the result of a failed induction.

- Malpresentations, such as shoulder or brow.
- Prolapse of the umbilical cord.
- Antepartum haemorrhage, due to the placenta separating early.
- Placenta praevia – the placenta is located over the cervix.
- Disproportion – the baby is too big to fit through the pelvis.
- Severe intrauterine growth retardation – the baby is growing poorly.
- Multiple pregnancy – more than 2 babies.
- Very large baby.
- Fetal abnormality.

Caesarean operations are also sometimes suggested for the following conditions, although research supports vaginal births in these cases. The risks from the Caesarean have to be weighed against any potential gains for the baby.

- Breech.
- Previous Caesarean section.
- Twins.
- History of infertility.
- Previous neonatal death.
- Maternal age.

How is it done?

There are two types of Caesarean births:

Elective – a complication occurs during the pregnancy which indicates a vaginal birth is inadvisable.

Emergency – a complication arises during labour, which requires immediate action.

Types of anaesthesia:

Epidural: the most commonly used anaesthesia unless there is a real emergency. The mother will be awake during the operation and can see and hold her baby straight away, unless the baby's condition requires urgent treatment. With an epidural, suction noises and changing internal pressures and tugging (but no pain) may be felt as the baby emerges. See epidural section for details on how this is administered.

Spinal anaesthetic: similar to an epidural, but faster acting and of shorter duration. Used in emergency situations as an alternative to an epidural. Further details below.

General anaesthetic: used if an emergency develops requiring immediate operation. The mother will be completely unconscious.

The specific procedures involved in a caesarean are as follows:

- The pubic hair is shaved and the area cleansed.
- A catheter is passed into the bladder to keep it empty.
- An intravenous drip line will be set up into the back of a hand.
- A blood pressure cuff is attached to give a continuous reading.
- The area will be surrounded with sterile drapes, and a drape will be erected as a screen so the operating area is out of sight of the mother.
- If the anaesthetic is to be an epidural or spinal time, is taken to ensure that it is completely effective.
- If a general anaesthetic is being used the mother will become unconscious very quickly.
- When anaesthesia is complete, an incision is made through the lower abdominal wall usually on the 'bikini line'.
- The bladder is lifted back, and the uterus is opened.
- The amniotic fluid is sucked from around the baby after the membranes have been opened.
- The baby is lifted from within, sometimes using forceps if the head is tightly wedged in the pelvic cavity.
- If an epidural or spinal has been used, at this stage the baby can be seen emerging and the first cries will be heard. It may be possible to hold the baby.
- As the baby is being born, an injection of Syntometrine is given to help the placenta to separate. This is then lifted out, and the wound stitched.
- Following the surgery the mother is taken to the recovery area and the baby may be taken to the nursery for observation. Support people can go with the baby to make initial contact.

Effects on the mother

Advantages:

- A Caesarean may be necessary to save the life of the mother, or to get the baby born.
- A lower segment Caesarean is less prone to complications later, heals well and the scar becomes invisible. The caesarean operation itself does not preclude a later vaginal birth.
- The use of epidural or spinal anaesthetics make it possible for mothers to be awake and aware during the birth to see and hear the baby born. This greatly facilitates bonding and post-operative recovery.

Disadvantages:

- A Caesarean section doubles the risk of maternal mortality.
- Since a Caesarean is abdominal surgery there are risks of damage to other internal organs and blood vessels.
- Caesarean section carries a risk of infection, which may prolong the hospital stay, interfere with the establishment of breastfeeding and delay post operative recovery.
- Side effects of the anaesthetic used must be considered. See separate entries for details of epidural and spinal anaesthetics.
- Women have been shown to have lower fertility rates following Caesarean section.
- The mother who has been unable to deliver vaginally can feel very disappointed. Even though she is no less a mother, she will need comfort and support from those around her if she is to be able to accept this unexpected outcome to her pregnancy.
- Separation of mother and baby may be the usual practice after a Caesarean, although the time involved may vary according to hospital routine and the health of mother and baby. If the baby must stay in the nursery, the mother can be taken to the nursery in a wheelchair, to see and touch her newborn.

Effects on the baby

Advantages:

- On occasion, a Caesarean may be life-saving for the baby.
- A Caesarean may be less traumatic for the baby than a difficult vaginal delivery, especially if the baby's health is at all in question.

Disadvantages:

- Depending on the reason for the Caesarean, the baby may already be 'at risk', and therefore extra treatment and observation may be necessary.
- The baby may be adversely affected by the anaesthetic used.
- The baby may be accidentally cut as the incision is made.
- The baby born after an elective Caesarean may be premature, and is more likely to have difficulties with breathing because of the absence of the stress hormones produced by the baby during a normal labour.
- Early separation of the mother and baby may interfere with bonding.
- The baby is less likely to be breastfed during this period of separation.

Drugs in labour

There are a number of drugs that may be offered to women during labour to ease the pain of labour. Before accepting any drugs, consider their possible effects carefully, just as you would for any drug offered in pregnancy. A list of questions you should ask your caregiver is included in Preparing For Birth: Fathers.

All drugs cross the placenta and will have an effect on the baby which will vary according to how much drug is used and how long it is in the mother's system before the baby is born.

Before birth, the mother will metabolise and eliminate the drug from her own body as well as her baby's. After birth, the baby must undertake these processes itself and this can take some time (days) due to its immature liver and kidneys.

It is impossible to predict how drugs will affect either the mother or her unborn baby. Everyone has their own tolerances to drugs, with some people finding that they are very sensitive while others are not. If you have not been exposed to the drugs given in labour before you will not know how they may affect you. It is impossible to know how your unborn baby will react to exposure to these drugs during labour.

There are alternative ways to ease the pain in labour without using drugs, and these should be explored fully before drugs are accepted.

PETHIDINE

Pethidine is a narcotic drug similar to morphine and heroin (diamorphine) that is given as a sedative in labour. It is not a pain killing drug, but may ease the pain indirectly as the mother becomes sedated.

Dosage:
The drug is supplied in prepared doses and 100mg is the commonest size, although smaller doses may be available. It should be given according to body weight. Pethidine is usually prescribed by a doctor but given by the midwife, and if a smaller dose is requested by the mother, the midwife will have to consult the doctor before the dose can be varied. 75 mg would be required for an average man when being used for post-operative pain.
It may be possible to request a smaller dose to begin, on the basis that if this is not enough, more can be administered later. Once in the system it is impossible to remove the drug except by waiting for the woman's body to eliminate the drug through her liver and kidneys (about 6 hours in a pregnant woman).

Time lag:
10–20 minutes

Duration:
2–3 hours
Route administered: Usually by injection into the thigh or buttock. Sometimes via a drip, if one is in place.

When given:
During first stage, once labour is established. Should not be given if the birth is expected within 2 hours. Sometimes given for pain relief following Caesarean section.

Effects on the mother

Advantages:

- Sedates.
- Has a secondary effect as a muscle relaxant, which may lessen pain and reduce muscle tension, allowing faster dilatation.
- May reduce pain.

Disadvantages:

- Does not relieve the pain directly.
- Creates a 'high', with feelings of floating and light-headedness that makes concentration difficult.
- Some people are so sedated that drowsiness makes it difficult to cope with contractions.
- Nausea, vomiting and dizziness are all common side-effects. An additional drug to counteract these effects is usually mixed with the pethidine before injection.
- Depresses the mother's breathing rate, which can reduce oxygenation of the blood.
- If the sedation results in a more rapid rate of dilatation than was expected, the baby may be born with more of the drug in its system than was intended.
- Opiate drugs cause delayed emptying of the stomach, increasing the risks of aspiration syndrome, a serious complication, if a general anaesthetic becomes necessary.

Effects on the baby

Advantages:
None.

Disadvantages:

- Pethidine crosses the placental barrier and depresses the baby's respiratory centre. This will cause breathing difficulties for the baby if it is born when the drug is at a maximum dosage in its system (between 1 and 3 hours after the injection).
- An antidote to counteract the depressive effects on the baby can be given but this gives only temporary relief and the baby may still suffer breathing difficulties when the antidote wears off after a few hours.
- Increased likelihood of jaundice as the baby's immature system works to eliminate the drug (and its antidote, if given). It may take 4–5 days for the baby to eliminate most of this drug from its system.
- Separation of mother and baby if these problems are severe.
- Difficulties establishing breastfeeding due to a depressed suckling reflex.
- Research has demonstrated a potential link between exposure of some babies to pethidine during labour and their later development of an addiction to opiate drugs as teenagers.

Other drugs sometimes mixed with pethidine

These drugs are sometimes given in the same injection with pethidine or may be given separately:

Sparine: to help enhance the action of pethidine and further reduce muscle tension.

Stematil: to help counter the side effects of nausea and dizziness caused by pethidine.

Maxilon: to reduce nausea and vomiting.

NITROUS OXIDE AND OXYGEN (ENTONOX)

A combination of two gases, nitrous oxide and oxygen in provide pain relief. Many hospitals use a dispenser that allows the proportion of the gases to be varied within a given range.

Dosage:
The dosage is variable with the range from 30% nitrous oxide 70% oxygen to 70% nitrous oxide 30% oxygen. Entonox is a fixed proportion of 50% nitrous oxide and 50% oxygen.

Time lag:
15 seconds

Drugs in labour CONTINUED

Duration:
Only effective whilst being breathed, plus about 15 seconds longer.
Route administered:
Via a face mask, which the mother holds tightly over her mouth and nose. Deep breathing is required to activate the dispensing machine, which can then be heard making a gurgling noise. It is important to start using the mask as soon as a contraction is felt to obtain the maximum effect. The mask should be taken off the face between contractions.
A mouthpiece may be available as an alternative to the face mask.
When given:
Usually during the transition phase of labour.
Effects on the mother
Advantages:
- An effective means of easing the pain, especially for the long and strong contractions of transition.
- Extra oxygen can be beneficial.
- Provides a distraction and a focus for attention during the turbulence of transition.

Disadvantages:
- Nausea and vomiting can be side effects.
- May make the mother drowsy and confused.
- Some women find the face mask unpleasant, even claustrophobic.
- Does not relieve the pain entirely.

Effects on the baby
Advantages:
- Extra oxygen could be beneficial.

Disadvantages:
- Research has shown a potential link between exposure of some babies to nitrous oxide during birth and their later development of an addiction to amphetamines as teenagers.

Anaesthetic drugs can be given by injection to relieve pain during labour.
An anaesthetist is required to administer an epidural or spinal anaesthetic. Obstetricians and GPs can give pudendal blocks and doctors or midwives may give local anaesthetics.

Anaesthetic injections

EPIDURAL ANAESTHETIC
An injection of local anaesthetic into the epidural space around the spinal cord which numbs the body below the injection site and thus relieves the pain from contractions.
It is the preferred anaesthetic for a woman having a Caesarean section, in which case the anaesthetic is injected into the spine a little higher up to give more widespread numbness.
Route administered:
A small amount of local anaesthetic, usually bupivacaine, is injected into the space around the spinal cord in between the third and fourth lumbar vertebrae. This may be done once then topped up at regular intervals, or may be delivered continuously through a special pump.
Dosage:
If full strength anaesthetic is used then the numbness will be complete and the mother will be unable to move her lower limbs, as the nerves supplying the muscles to the legs will be completely anaesthetised.
Low dose epidurals use a half or quarter strength dose, and this will numb sensation and remove the pain of the contractions whilst not affecting the nerve supply to muscles. The mother will be able to move her legs and sit up, whilst not feeling any sensation.
Sometimes, the low dose of local anaesthetic is mixed with Pethidine or Fentanyl (a similar opiate) allowing less of each drug to be used, while still giving good pain relief. Greater mobility and fewer side effects are also reported.
Time lag:
Between 5 and 15 minutes from injection.
Duration:
About 3 hours for a full strength anaesthetic, proportionally less for low dose epidurals.

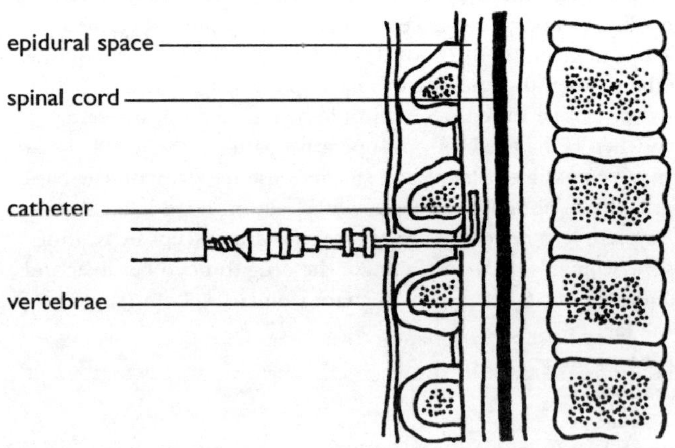

When given:
- For pain relief, at any time in first stage, but usually once labour is fully established.
- Prior to a Caesarean section.
- To reduce high blood pressure during labour.

Effects on the mother
Advantages:
- A usually reliable method of pain relief, with complete loss of sensation from the waist down.
- Can help to control high blood pressure.
- Facilitates a forceps delivery if complications are present.

- Allows the mother to be conscious during a Caesarean section.
- Relief from pain may allow greater relaxation and more rapid dilatation.
- Relieving the pain may increase the mother's positive feelings about labour and birth.

Disadvantages:

- The mother will be confined to bed, with resultant loss of mobility. If the dosage is half or quarter strength, she may be able to sit up, even move around, if well supported.
- In 10–15% of cases, the anaesthetic may not take completely leaving some areas not fully anaesthetised.
- Administration of an epidural slows the labour down so that oxytocic drugs may be needed to keep contractions going.
- The mother's blood pressure can fall dramatically following an epidural and this is sometimes used as a reason for using an epidural. A drip will always be inserted prior to epidural administration in case treatment for low blood pressure becomes necessary.
- There is an increased likelihood that the mother's temperature will rise the longer an epidural is in place. If this happens the baby's temperature will also rise, increasing the risk of fetal distress.
- It may be difficult to empty the bladder and a catheter is frequently necessary.
- In inexperienced hands, the covering of the spinal cord may be punctured. This will result in a leaking of spinal fluid and the mother will have a severe headache (perhaps for several days) until the puncture wound heals and the leaking stops. It may be possible to repair the leak by injecting a small amount of the woman's own blood into the epidural space. As this clots, it forms a patch over the hole, sealing it from further leaks. If successful, the headache will disappear almost immediately.
- The muscles of the pelvic floor are relaxed by the anaesthetic and as a result the baby's head is less likely to rotate, and a forceps delivery may be necessary.
- With a full strength epidural, the mother will feel no urge to push unless it is allowed to wear off before second stage commences. Forceps may be needed to lift the baby out.
- The mother will have a reduced sensation of giving birth to her baby.
- Tenderness over the area where the needle was inserted is common in the days following birth.
- There is an absence of tone in the muscles that support the lower vertebrae and sacroiliac joints especially with a full epidural in place. This causes lack of stability in the joints, and moving the mother may cause them to become misaligned, leading to chronic backache that may last weeks or months following the birth.
- If the baby is affected by the drugs, the mother may perceive her baby as 'difficult' and hard to settle, making breastfeeding and nurturing more difficult. This perception can persist for some months.
- Paraplegia is a very, very rare but unpredictable complication.

Effects on the baby

Advantages:

- The mother will be able to make immediate contact following a Caesarean section, and may be able to breastfeed.
- Reduced risk of fetal distress if the mother's high blood pressure can be reduced.
- The mother may feel more positive about labour, birth and the baby if she is free of pain.

Disadvantages:

- The baby will be affected by the drugs used, depending on the length of their exposure before birth. Common reactions include irritability, an inability to settle easily and a tendency to startle easily. These effects may last several weeks.
- If any obstetric complications occur as a result of the epidural, these will have additional side effects on the baby.
- Should further intervention become necessary, such as an oxytocin drip, forceps, vacuum extraction, episiotomy or Caesarean section, the baby will be affected by these procedures. See separate entries for summaries.
- Any obstetric intervention or complication increases the likelihood of separation of mother and baby in the early post-natal period.

SPINAL ANALGESIA

A quick acting anaesthetic useful for emergency use for Caesarean section.

Route administered:

A procedure similar to an epidural, except that the injection of anaesthetic is into the spinal cord itself.

Dosage:

Only one tenth of the amount of anaesthetic (bupivacaine) is necessary compared to an epidural. Sometimes is it mixed with either pethidine or fentanyl. It is given as 'one-shot' procedure (not topped up regularly).

Time lag:

Anaesthesia is usually achieved within 5 minutes.

Duration:

Lasts between 75 and 120 minutes.

When given:

- For Caesarean section, especially in an emergency situation if an epidural is not already in place.
- For elective Caesarean sections.
- When the placenta needs to be removed manually.

Effects on the mother

Advantages

- A quick acting anaesthetic in an emergency situation.
- A very reliable form of anaesthetic, with very low failure rate in experienced hands.
- Uses less anaesthetic, so reduces the risk of side effects.
- Reduced risk of headache, as a very fine needle is used.

Disadvantages

- Requires an experienced anaesthetist as it is a more technically difficult procedure.
- Risk of a severe headache if several attempts are needed for successful placement.
- Unable to be topped up if the anaesthesia proves inadequate. Other pain-killing drugs may have to be given in addition, or a general anaesthetic.
- Too much anaesthetic may cause a profound drop in blood pressure which will require prompt treatment.
- Nausea and vomiting may occur.

Effects on the baby

Advantages

- May enable the baby to be born faster in an emergency.
- Less exposure to drugs than for epidural anaesthetics.

Disadvantages

- The baby may be affected by the drugs used.
- A sudden drop in blood pressure may lead to fetal distress.
- If any complication occurs as a result of the procedure (such as the need for a general anaesthetic), this may have effects on the baby.

PUDENDAL BLOCK

This is an injection of local anaesthetic into the perineal area to numb the outlet.

Route administered:

The anaesthetic is injected through the walls of the vagina into the nerves on both sides of the vagina. This deadens the whole of the pelvic outlet.

Time lag:

The anaesthetic will take effect immediately.

Duration:

The area should stay numb long enough to enable any necessary stitching to be done after the birth.

When given:

At the beginning of second stage.

Effects on the mother

Advantages:

- Numbs the perineum.
- Allows an early episiotomy.
- Allows a pain-free birth.

Disadvantages:

- Reduces the urge to push, which may delay second stage or require the use of forceps.
- The mother cannot feel the baby being born.
- If an early episiotomy is done, then extensive bruising of tissues and blood loss will occur.

Effects on the baby

Advantages:

- The baby may be born faster if episiotomy is done.

Disadvantages:

- The baby may be affected by exposure to the anaesthetic.

LOCAL ANAESTHESIA OF THE PERINEUM

Local anaesthetic is usually injected into the perineum before an episiotomy is performed. If the episiotomy is done when the area is somewhat numb from stretching, then the anaesthetic may not be needed. It will be given prior to stitching the wound. If the mother tears during the birth the area will be anaesthetised before stitching occurs.

Route administered:

A series of small injections are made into the area where the cut will be made or where the stitches will be placed.

Time lag:

Immediate effect.

Duration:

The area will stay anaesthetised long enough to allow the stitching to be done.

When given:

During second stage prior to performing an episiotomy. After the birth, prior to stitching up the wound or tear.

Effects on the mother

Advantages:

- Numbs the area so that the episiotomy will not be felt.
- Numbs the area so that the stitching will be pain-free.

Disadvantages:

- The injections can be painful.

Effects on the baby

Advantages:

- The baby will not receive any appreciable amount of drug because the birth is imminent.

Disadvantages:

- The baby may be affected by exposure to the anaesthetic.

After the baby is born

After the baby is born

Your new baby

Your baby will look like an individual right from the start. You may be surprised at its appearance, and perhaps puzzled by some of the characteristics most babies show. Some examples follow.

Some babies are born with blue bodies and faces. As the baby begins to breathe oxygen from the air, it will quickly turn pink. Sometimes it takes a little longer for the hands and feet to be completely pink, but this is normal and will improve as the circulation quickly improves.

The baby's head is large in proportion to the body, with a button nose and a receding chin. These help the baby to latch on to the breast. The eyes are usually grey and will change in a few months to their final colour.

Larger babies are more chubby, and have a layer of fat underneath the skin which gives them a rounded look (and adds to their weight). Premature or smaller babies usually have little body fat at birth.

The skin may be slightly dry, and even flaky in the creases. There may be a layer of vernix, a cheesy white substance, which provides protection for the baby's skin while immersed in the amniotic fluid. The vernix can be left on or gently massaged into the skin.

Fingernails are often long and very soft. If the baby keeps scratching his face, cut the nails with small scissors.

Genitalia appear very large at birth. Little boys can have erections right from birth, and little girls sometimes menstruate slightly as the baby adjusts to the absence of the mother's hormones. Breasts of both boys and girls may be swollen and secrete fluid at first. This is normal and will pass of its own accord in a few days.

Most babies will have some degree of moulding of the head at birth, due to the pressure as it passes through the pelvis. This usually disappears within 24–48 hours.

If the mother has not needed drugs during the labour, the baby will be alert and wide eyed. Not all babies cry lustily after birth – some just want to look around and take everything in. Whilst your baby is awake and peaceful, take the time to cuddle and breastfeed. These first moments are very precious.

If the mother needed drugs during labour, the baby may be drowsy, sleepy or irritable after the birth. Reactions vary, and you should realise that this is a passing phase, and within a few days your baby will have excreted the drugs and be showing more normal behaviour. If your baby is irritable, try to comfort as best you can. If the baby is sleepy, don't allow him to sleep too long between feeds as the baby needs colostrum for food and protection from infection, and also to help in the elimination of the drugs.

CARE OF THE NEWBORN BABY

During the days following birth, a number of checks will be made to ensure that your baby is healthy and progressing well. These tests may be carried out by the midwife, or in some cases, by a paediatrician. All of them can be done in your presence so you know what is being done, and can ask appropriate questions.

First examination

Soon after birth, a number of basic observations will be made, including generally noting its appearance, breathing, colour, heart beat, muscle tone and reflexes. These will be recorded as the APGAR score. The weight will be recorded and its body length and head circumference noted.

Vitamin K

Vitamin K is essential for the normal clotting of blood and it is made in the body from the food we eat. Babies are born with almost no Vitamin K in their system and it is not known why nature has provided this arrangement. To protect the baby from the possible hazards of bleeding, especially if the birth was traumatic or premature (with the baby requiring treatments), an injection of Vitamin K is usually offered within hours of the birth. The vitamin can also be given orally.

After a few days, the baby will have manufactured sufficient Vitamin K in its body from the breastmilk to give an adequate level of clotting factor in its blood.

SCREENING TESTS

There are a variety of tests that may be done in the first few days to detect any abnormalities. Screening tests are designed to identify those babies who may have a problem requiring further investigation – they are not diagnostic tests themselves. Screening tests include:

Guthrie test

This checks for the presence of a rare condition called phenylketonuria (PKU) a potentially serious disease caused by the lack of an enzyme which is necessary for the assimilation of amino acids in protein foods.

The test must be carried out after the baby has been exposed to the protein in milk and is usually done on the fifth day after birth. Blood is obtained from a heel prick and processed within a few days.

The same blood can also be tested for:
Cystic fibrosis – a condition where all the endocrine systems are affected and the secretory organs becomes blocked. Physiotherapy can help.

Hypothyroidism – an early diagnosis can facilitate control with thyroid tablets.

Galactosaemia – the enzyme which digests galactose is absent and the baby must have a galactose-free diet.

Tests for hip stability
The baby's hip joints will be manipulated to help diagnose any problems with congenital dislocation. Early treatment ensures good outcomes.

CIRCUMCISION

This is the surgical removal of the skin over the tip of the penis, usually carried out within the first few days after birth. As it is not safe to give anaesthetics to newborns, the procedure is done without any anaesthetic.

Unless there is a religious reason or deformity (which makes the passing of urine difficult), doctors are agreed that circumcision is unnecessary, and carries risks of infection and poor surgical technique.

If you decide against circumcision, it is important to know that the foreskin is normally adherent to the tip of the penis until the second or third year, and that forcible retraction of the foreskin can lead to infection and other complications. When the skin is ready to retract it will do so, probably as a result of the boy's own explorations. In the meantime, general hygiene is all that is required.

Learning to breastfeed

Breastfeeding is the ideal way to continue the close relationship you have formed with your baby during the pregnancy, and the ideal source of nourishment, adapted to his specific needs. You will find there are many advantages, from ease of portability and constant availability, to the regular rest periods and extended physical contact that breastfeeding ensures. It is time-saving and cheap, gives protection from illness, and helps you to regain your figure.

Breastfeeding should begin as soon as possible after the birth. If, due to illness of the baby or mother, the first feed has to be delayed, be patient and follow the same steps as other mothers when you are able to begin nursing.

If your baby is born prematurely, your milk will have extra protein to help him catch up, and the antibacterial and immunological factors he needs to avoid infection and fight disease. If the baby can't suck strongly because he is too little, express your milk and feed it via tube or eye-dropper. The sucking urge will develop as he grows.

THE FIRST HOUR AFTER BIRTH

Putting the baby to the breast is really part of the birth process, as the nipple stimulation causes the uterus to contract, which helps the placenta to separate and be expelled.

The suckling response of the baby is strongest in the first hour, and the nipples are extraordinarily sensitive. This combination means that even if the first nursing is not for very long or even very successful, the uterus will respond. The baby will have his first sucking efforts rewarded through tasting his first colostrum. If there is a delay in putting the baby to the breast, or the baby is lethargic due to labour drugs, try again as soon as you can.

POSITIONING THE BABY

Holding the baby so that the nipple is grasped at the correct angle will make breastfeeding easy and avoid many common problems. For the first feed after birth, unwrap the baby a little so his hands are free and skin-to-skin contact can be achieved. This will keep him warm and make positioning easier. Place him along your arm, with your hand under his nappy or bottom, and his head lying in the crook of your elbow – don't hold his head. Make sure his tummy is against your stomach, and that he is lying on his side. He should have one arm under your breast, the other free to move on top. His head, neck and spine should be in a straight line (his head should not be turned to the side). You will find all this easier if you sit upright, with a pillow behind your back and another under the arm supporting the baby.

Learning to breastfeed CONTINUED

Raise or lower the baby until his nose is opposite the nipple, tucking his feet in close against your body. Check that the nipple is erect, and if not gently massage it to a good shape. Allow the baby time to explore and lick the nipple and, as he opens his mouth wide, pull him towards you using your whole arm. The nipple should go into the back of his mouth, and he will easily latch on. His chin should be firmly pressed into the underside of your breast and his nose free so he can breathe. If necessary use your free hand to support the breast. The areola (the dark area around the nipple) should be under his lips, which are flared back in an open-mouthed position.

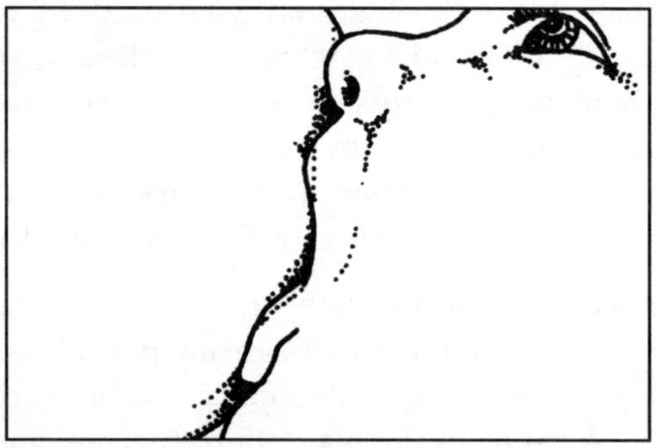

If you don't get him well positioned, release his suction by putting your finger in the corner of his mouth and try again.

Allow him to empty the first breast, then switch him over to the second side to finish off. Alternate the breast you start with each time. If he is well positioned, your nipples will not become cracked or sore, apart from a little initial tenderness as they adjust to the nursing process.

ROUTINE IN HOSPITAL

It is important to feed your baby according to need, both yours and his. Most newborns will need to be fed every 3 hours, and you need to feed at night to avoid engorged breasts. Time at the breast need not be restricted unless the nipples are very sore or cracked, when attention to correct positioning should be given first.

It is not necessary to give any extra fluids to the baby. The colostrum, the first milk produced in your breasts, is an especially rich milk and will help the baby to avoid jaundice and maintain body weight. Most babies will settle more easily if with their mothers, so full rooming-in, especially at night is an advantage. Having the baby in bed will help calm a fractious baby and thereby allow the mother more sleep.

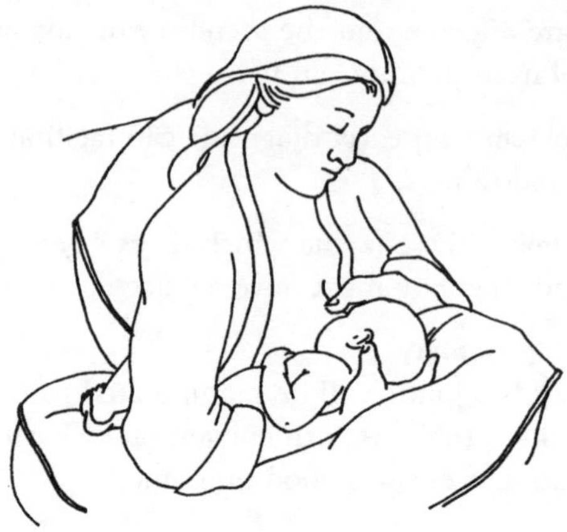

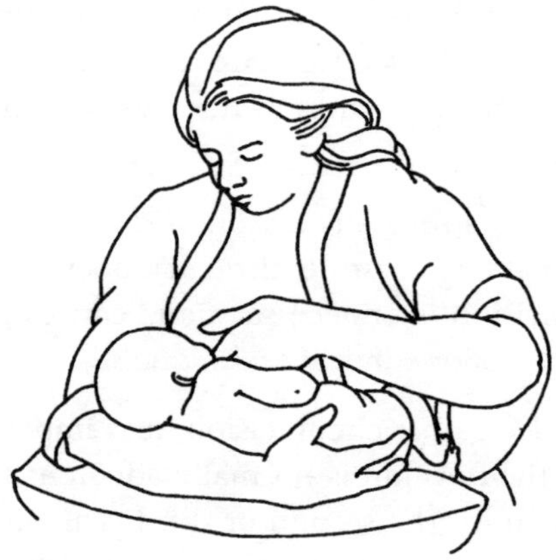

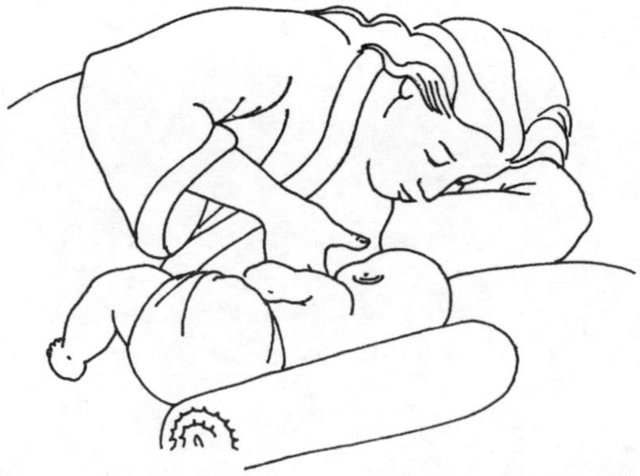

There is more than one way to hold the baby when nursing. Experiment to find a comfortable position for you and the baby.

Learning to breastfeed CONTINUED

OVERCOMING EARLY BREASTFEEDING PROBLEMS
If you experience problems with breastfeeding, or nursing is painful, seek advice from a knowledgeable midwife, community breastfeeding counsellor or Lactation Consultant.

Sore nipples are usually caused by poor positioning and can be helped by attention to this together with varying nursing positions, drying the nipples and limited suckling time. Sore nipples can also be caused by thrush infection in the baby's mouth transferring to the nipple area, and this may require treatment.

Engorgement usually occurs as the milk comes in around the third day. The breasts fill up and become hard and painful. It can also be caused by omitting night feeds, or allowing long time lapses between feeds. Hand expression before the feed will soften the breast, help the baby to latch on and ease any lumps that may be forming.

A poor supply of milk can easily be improved through increased feeding. It takes six weeks to establish lactation, which operates on a supply = demand basis. The more often your baby asks to be fed, the more milk you will make to satisfy his needs.

The let-down reflex is the mechanism employed by the body to get the milk to the baby. It is sometimes seen as milk squirting or dripping from the breasts or felt as a tingling sensation at the beginning of the feed. This shows that your milk is flowing well to the baby.

JAUNDICE
Most babies become a little jaundiced in the first few days, as their bodies eliminate excess bilirubin from their bloodstream. If your baby appears more yellow than normal, a blood test will be done to estimate the level of jaundice. It may be necessary to expose the baby to extra light from fluorescent tubes in an incubator to help him eliminate the excess bilirubin. This may take a few hours or days, if severe. During this time, his eyes will be covered, and he will be sleepy.

Continue to feed him as often as you can, even though he may be sleepy at the breast. The breastmilk will help him obtain the fluids he needs at this time.

Your post-partum recovery

Following the birth of your baby, your body will gradually return to its pre-pregnant state. This will take several months. In the first few weeks however, you will notice the following:

LOCHIA
You will have some bleeding following the birth, and it will be red at first, then turn a reddish-brown, then finally, after about 2 weeks, become a clear discharge. The lochia usually disappears after 3–4 weeks. The initial bleeding will be most noticeable when you breastfeed, as the uterus contracts at this time. If bleeding persists, mention it to your doctor at the six week check-up. If you suddenly bleed very heavily, go to the hospital immediately, as you may be having a haemorrhage caused by some remnants of the placenta or membranes still inside your uterus.

If the lochia takes time to clear, increase your intake of iron to counteract any tendency to anaemia which will cause excessive tiredness.

AFTERBIRTH PAINS
When you breastfeed your baby, the release of oxytocin in response to nipple stimulation causes the uterus to contract. In the first few days these contractions can be unpleasant, especially if this is not your first baby, and the resultant pain can be difficult to cope with. These pains usually become less severe with each passing day, and although a nuisance, they indicate that your uterus is returning to its pre-pregnant size. Try deep breathing and relaxation as you settle down to nurse your baby and applying a hot pack (e.g. a hot water bottle) to the area may help. If this is not enough, some paracetamol (Panadol) taken about hour before a feed in the first few days will help you cope.

STITCHES
If you have needed stitches following the birth, these hints may help ease the discomfort until they have healed:

- Do your pelvic floor exercises as soon as you can. These will help improve circulation and speed the healing process.
- The first few times you have your bowels open, hold a pad against your perineum. This will help you protect the stitched area and stop the feeling that you are tearing apart (which won't happen).
- Lie on your side to feed the baby.
- Use an air ring when sitting in bed or on a chair.
- Warm baths from time to time are soothing.

- Keep the area dry as much as you can, as this promotes healing.

Report any swelling, bruising or anything you may think is even slightly abnormal to the midwives. Stitches should have healed by 3 weeks. If this has not occurred, see a doctor or midwife and have them checked.

If your perineal area is still uncomfortable when you have your six-week check-up, tell your midwife or doctor, and seek treatment.

The first few times you have sexual intercourse, use a lubricating jelly. You may need to experiment with alternative positions for comfort too.

"THIRD DAY BLUES"

Some women feel weepy and emotional several days after the birth. This is usually a temporary state and is a passing phase as your body returns to normal hormonal levels. Having a good cry often helps. True post-natal depression is more common after several weeks, when a feeling of apathy and lethargy develops, perhaps coupled with anxiety or nervousness. If you start feeling like this alert you partner or a friend so that appropriate help and support can be obtained.

CONTRACEPTION

You need to consider using contraception as soon as you want to resume having sex. Many women want to delay this until the six week check-up but you need not wait that long if any stitches have healed and you feel ready. If you have had a Caesarean, you will want to wait until the scar is comfortably healed. If you are breastfeeding, you will find that vaginal dryness may be a problem at first, due to your changed levels of hormones and a low oestrogen level. Use some lubrication and take it very gently the first few times.

If you are not breastfeeding you will have your first period usually 4–6 weeks after the baby is born. If you are breastfeeding, ovulation is likely to be delayed some time, but as soon as your baby starts sleeping longer at night, takes food other that breastmilk or spaces his feeds to more than 3 hours, then you are more likely to resume ovulation. To be absolutely safe, you need to decide as soon as the baby is born to use contraception, even though a breastfeeding mother may have months before ovulation begins again.

The non-breastfeeding mother can use any of the contraceptives available, although the IUD should not be fitted before 8 weeks to allow time for the uterus to return to its normal size. The contraceptive pill can be started straight after the birth. The diaphragm will need to be checked for fit by your midwife or doctor following birth.

For the breastfeeding mother, the range of contraceptives is more limited.

The 'mini pill' (progestogen only pill) is often prescribed, although the manufacturers state it should not be used by breastfeeding mothers. It works by thickening the cervical mucous and changing the lining of the uterus to make implantation of a fertilised egg difficult, so it must be taken at the same time each day, preferably at least 4 hours before having sex. Some women find that they become irritable or depressed on this pill, and that their milk supply is affected.

Most IUDs that remain on the market contain copper, and because this can build up in the lining of the uterus until menstruation resumes, there is concern that this may be harmful to mother and baby (via the breastmilk). As yet, there has been no scientific work done to explore this possibility, but it might be wise to delay using an IUD until the periods resume.

Diaphragms need to be refitted after having a baby and also if there is much change in body-weight in the following months. They are reliable if used properly and with a spermicide. If you have not used one before, make sure you are shown how to insert it when you are fitted.

Condoms are a simple alternative. Lubrication may be needed if the vagina is dry.

Natural family planning methods are difficult to learn while you are breastfeeding and periods are absent or irregular. To be successful, you must learn the method from a fully qualified counsellor, who will teach you the signs of fertility and show you how to record them.

Sterilisation by tubal ligation or vasectomy can be considered if your family is complete. Before embarking on either of these alternatives, you will need counselling and a full explanation of the techniques used.

It is recommended that you discuss contraception with your midwife or doctor at the six week check-up or with a Family Planning Association counsellor soon after the birth. If you are breastfeeding, you need to consider yourself and the baby when you make your choice. If the method you choose doesn't suit you or you have unpleasant side-effects, change to another method, again seeking guidance if necessary.

Your post-partum recovery CONTINUED

FATIGUE

The most common problem facing every new mother is fatigue. Broken sleep, natural anxiety about baby care and well being and hurried or skimpy meals contribute to tiredness, which can effect your enjoyment of the baby and interfere with your relationship with your partner.

In the first few weeks, make time each day to have a rest, to compensate for lost sleep at night. Feed the baby lying down and doze afterwards for as long as you can. Try to make night feeds quicker by avoiding nappy changing (and disturbing or waking the baby) unless absolutely necessary. Try to limit visitors to times when you have extra help available so you won't miss out on your daily nap.

Make sure that your diet is adequate. Cook up extra servings whenever possible so you have ready made meals for busy times or lunches. Eat nourishing snacks, such as boiled eggs, cheese sticks, fruit, cold cooked chicken, wholemeal bread. An afternoon snack containing whole-grain with some fruit and a glass of milk will provide energy for the hectic time in the evening, when most babies are awake and sometimes irritable.

ROUTINES

It is really impossible to have any kind of routine in the first few months with a new baby. Gradually a pattern will emerge, but it will take perhaps as long as twelve months for regular sleep times etc to develop. In the meantime, take your cues from the baby and respond to his needs, rather than trying to get him to conform to your desired routines. When the baby is happy, everyone else will be happy too. It helps to reassess priorities in housework to eliminate unnecessary chores. It is more worthwhile to spend time with your baby either playing or cuddling than having a spotless house, and you'll find that eventually the baby will need less attention and you can give the house some extra care.

GETTING HELP

If you have a baby who cries a lot, is hard to settle or sleeps very little, it is helpful to be able to call on others for support or advice. Your local Early Childhood Nurse or Health Visitor will have names of local mothers' groups, breastfeeding support groups, or playgroups. Talking to other mothers is a big help and very reassuring. There are also a number of good books that will reassure you and assist with suggestions. Especially useful are the 'how to' breastfeeding books, which can offer consistent advice about breastfeeding problems.

FOR THE FATHERS

Although most of this section has been directed towards the mother of your baby, your role is vital and you will find much pleasure from nurturing your relationship with your baby and partner. You need to allow yourself time to spend with the baby, not just to ease the burden on your partner, but to discover for yourself the special qualities and personality of your baby. Babies love the different 'feel' of their fathers - the strong hands, deep voice and the different games they play. Participating in the daily routine of baby care is not a waste of time or unmanly, but a special opportunity for interaction with your child.

Your partner will need time to adjust to her new role as a mother and to physically revert to her non-pregnant state. If she breastfeeds, her primary focus of attention must be the baby, but this does not mean that she doesn't want a close relationship with you too. Explore new ways of being tender and close, and accept that this is just a phase that will pass as your child grows and no longer needs her total attention.

Support and encouragement from you will be appreciated by her at this time. It is a time of learning for you both, a special time in your lives and a great opportunity for learning more about yourselves as people. Try not to rush or ignore it.

Savour and enjoy!

Post-natal exercises

As soon as your baby is born you can begin gentle exercises to help you get back into shape.

You can begin these exercises from the first day after the birth, but it will take from six months to a year to regain your figure completely. Breastfeeding (to help you lose extra weight gained in pregnancy) and a general exercise program of walking, swimming or suitable aerobics will also help, after the first few weeks.

Pelvic floor exercises

These can be started right after the birth and are especially important because the pelvic floor muscles have been considerably stretched during the birth. If you have stitches or haemorrhoids, exercise to the point of discomfort. Doing these exercises will help reduce swelling and restore the supportive muscles underneath, useful aids to increased comfort. The pelvic floor exercises are the same as those practised in pregnancy see page 13 for details.

Each time you pick the baby up, cough or have to lift anything, tighten the pelvic floor and lower abdominal muscles first. This will enable you to exercise the muscles regularly.

Pelvic rocking

This is a simple exercise that will help relieve backache. Lie on your back and tighten your abdominal muscles as you flatten your lower spine against the floor. Release. Repeat several times in succession.

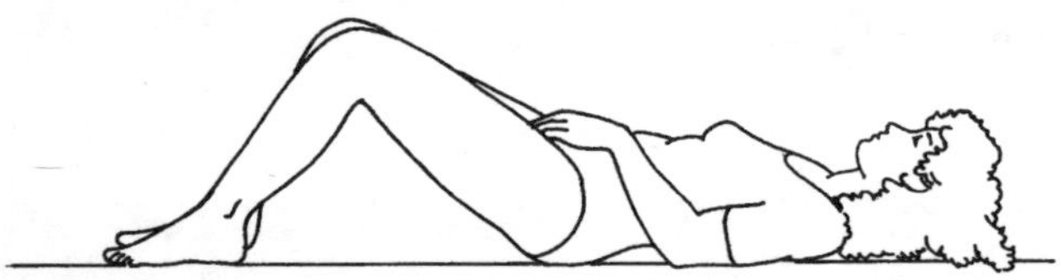

Tummy tucking

Sitting on a chair, pull in your tummy muscles below your belly button, as though you are trying to make them touch your spine. Repeat several times, holding for a few seconds each time. Do this often, and also in preparation for lifting objects or getting up from a chair.

Before beginning more strenuous abdominal exercises, check that the abdominal muscles between the lower ribs and the pubic bone have come together. These muscles have to stretch to allow the baby to grow, and after the birth remain slightly apart. You should wait until you can only insert the tips of two fingers in the space between them while you raise your head from the pillow. This will take about 8 weeks following the birth.

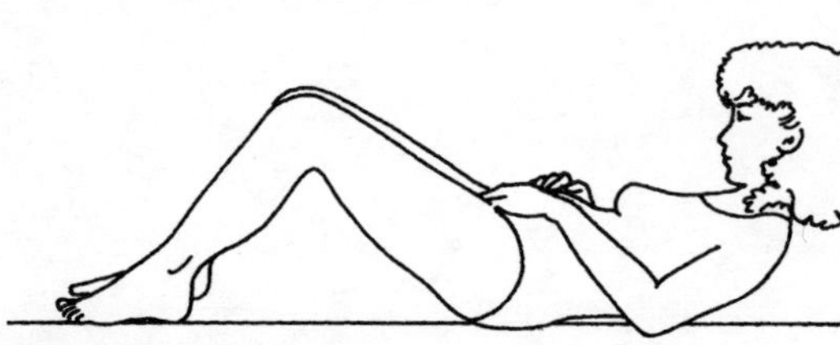

Raise your head and shoulders to reach across your body to the outside of one knee. Hold briefly then release. Do the opposite side, breathing out as you reach up and in as you release.

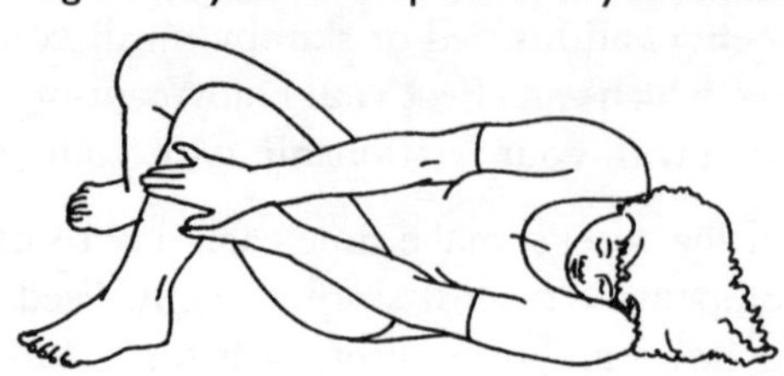

Exercising with baby

When you are ready for stronger exercise, include the baby it is fun for you both and can form part of your daily play time.

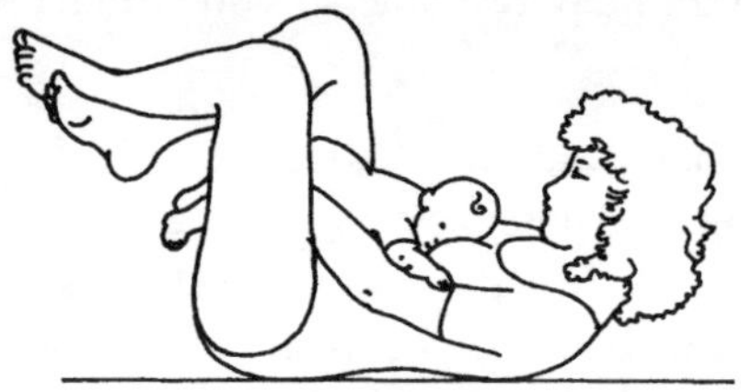

Lie your baby on your tummy and raise your head and shoulders whilst bringing your knees to your chest. Rest with your feet off the floor. Repeat up to ten times. When you have finished lower one foot first, then the other.

Sit your baby on your pubic bone supported by your legs. Hold on to baby's chest as you circle around with your legs. Raise your head and shoulders at the same time.

Lie the baby across your lower legs. Lift your shoulders and head and talk to the baby. Keeping your head up, extend your legs as far as you can. Keep your back flat against the floor while you do this exercise.

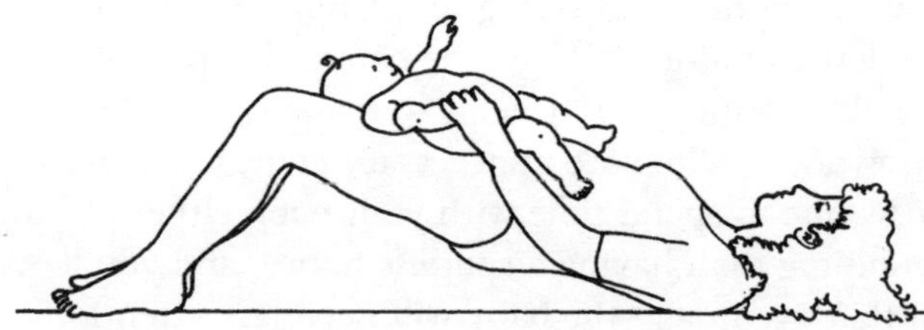

Lie the baby along your legs. Tighten your buttocks and pelvic floor and lift your hips up slowly until they form a straight line with your back and shoulders. Unroll gradually.

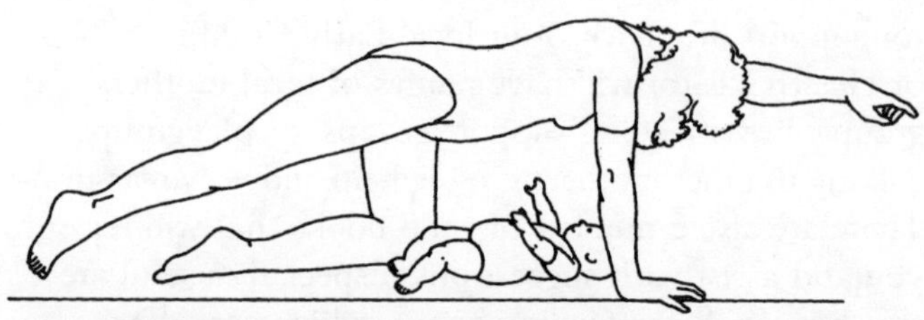

Lie the baby on the floor. Starting on hands and knees, extend one arm and the opposite leg, no higher than the level of the hip. Change over, and exercise the other arm and leg.

Class Evaluation

Being very conscious of the need to maintain a high standard of teaching, your prenatal educator would appreciate you taking time to fill out this assessment. Please return it to your educator after your baby has arrived. Your comments will help your educator to review class content, and is one way to ensure that the needs of class members are being met.

Please fill in the blanks and circle the answers that apply:

Educators's name

....

Date of class series

....

Your name and address (optional)

....

....

....

Filled in by

Mother Father Both

1. How would you describe your fears and anxieties about childbirth before you took these classes?
   great moderate minimal none
2. Now that you have completed the classes, how would you describe your attitudes?
   more positive more negative about the same
3. Any topics that should have been included?

   ....

   ....
4. Any topics that should have been left out?

   ....

   ....
5. Should there have been more time devoted to any topic? Please list these:

   ....

   ....

   ....

   ....
6. Was ample time allotted for (answer Yes or No):

   review

   practice

   questions
7. Did you find the information presented in class to be:
   usually too deep too superficial at a good level
8. In general, the classes were (circle as many as apply):
   interesting boring exciting tedious alarming
   comfortable relaxing stimulating

   other (specify)
9. The teacher presented information in a manner which was:
   positive inflexible encouraging threatening
   friendly indifferent relaxed supportive
   objective balanced subjective

   other (specify)
10. The most important part of the class was:

    ....

    ....
11. The thing you enjoyed least was:

    ....

    ....
12. Any other comments?

    ....

    ....

    ....

Please photocopy or tear out and send to your educator (or her employer), whose name and address is:

Your birth experience

Your educator would appreciate having some details of your birth experience to assist when explaining birth options and variations in labour to other parents. Please complete this questionnaire and return it as soon as you can after the birth (before you forget the details yourself!)

Your name (optional)

Hospital

Midwife or Doctor

Date when your baby was born

Weight

Length

Sex ☐ Male ☐ Female

Is this your ☐ first ☐ second ☐ (other) baby?

How long was your labour?

How many days before or after your due date did labour start?

days before

days after

Did any complications occur during labour or birth? Please tick:

- ☐ premature
- ☐ fetal distress
- ☐ forceps
- ☐ Caesarean section
- ☐ induction
- ☐ episiotomy

Do you have any on-going discomforts from the birth?

Did you receive any of the following?

☐ electronic fetal monitoring, when

☐ pethidine: mg

☐ epidural, given because

Full strength, half strength?

☐ pudendal block, given because

☐ Gas mask

☐ oxytocin drip, given because

Were the advantages and disadvantages of these procedures explained to you at the time?

Were you able to labour in a shower or bath?

What position did you use for giving birth:

- ☐ standing
- ☐ kneeling
- ☐ squatting
- ☐ side lying
- ☐ on all fours
- ☐ flat on your back
- ☐ legs in stirrups
- ☐ semi-sitting
- ☐ on a mat on the floor
- ☐ birth stool
- ☐ under water
- ☐ on the bed

If you were induced, what was the reason given?

The membranes:

broke on their own, at

were broken by the midwife/doctor when

Did you hold the baby immediately after the birth? Y / N

For how long?

When did you first breastfeed your baby?

Please use an extra page to describe your labour, including the birth and the time in hospital. Include any details you would like to share about the hospital care, your caregiver or the time afterwards. Many thanks for taking the time to tell us about your birth!